Health Controls Wealth

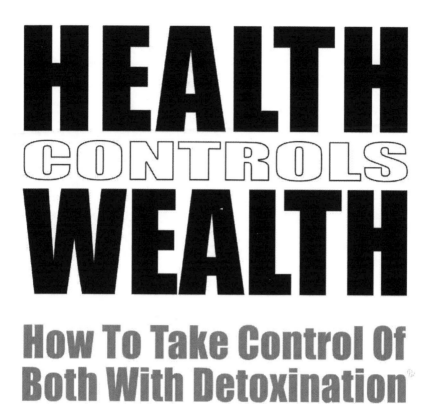

HEALTH CONTROLS WEALTH

How To Take Control Of Both With Detoxination

By

Daniel L. Root with David E. Root, M.D., M.P.H.

Disclaimer:

Information in this book is provided for educational purposes only. You may use the work for your own noncommercial and personal use; any other use of the work is strictly prohibited. The information is a result of years of clinical practice experience by the authors. This information is not intended as a substitute for the advice provided by your physician or other healthcare professional. Do not use the information in this book for diagnosing or treating a health problem or disease, or prescribing medication or other treatment. Always speak with your physician or other healthcare professional before taking any medication or nutritional, herbal or homeopathic supplement, or using any treatment for a health problem. If you have or suspect that you have a medical problem, contact your health care provider promptly. Do not disregard professional medical advice or delay in seeking professional advice because of something you have read in this book. Information provided here and the use of any products or services purchased from us by you does not *create a doctor-patient relationship between you and any of the physicians affiliated with our business. Information and statements regarding dietary supplements have not been evaluated by the Food and Drug Administration and are not intended to diagnose, treat, cure, or prevent any disease.*

DEDICATION

For my wonderful wife and inspiration, Suzy, for putting up with me throughout the many long hours developing the business and writing of this book.

And to my beautiful daughters, who forgave me for missing a soccer game or two, as well!

Table of Contents

FOREWORD

by Nenah Sylver, PhD

Body heating has existed for thousands of years. The Finns, passionate about sauna, sweated in cozy wooden shacks that doubled as smokehouses and occasionally birthing rooms. The Turks built massive, elaborate marble and brick hammans and sweated in style, sometimes adding steam. Mushi-buros, petite to match the Japanese who crawled into them, were molded from clay. In Mexico, the mortar temescals boasted statues of the Goddess of Sweat. In North America, the most well-known sweat chamber was the Native American sweat lodge. Many different tribes arranged long branches in cathedral-like arches, covered them with animal hides, and then filled the pit at the center of the enclosure with hot fired stones. These sweat lodges, like other places for sweating, were considered sacred. The purification that the occupants received was on all levels: physical, emotional, mental, and spiritual.

Today's modern saunas are built of wood, stone, clay, and plastic. The heaters have become highly sophisticated to match our technology—powered by gas and electricity, with variable settings, and often comprised of synthetic materials such as carbon and ceramic. However, the concept is the same. Sweat equals cleansing. But what, exactly, are we cleansing? And why do we need to do it?

In 2004, my search for answers led me to write the 360-page Holistic Handbook of Sauna Therapy. I explored the colorful history of saunas and its cousins, steam rooms and hydrotherapy. Readers were told how and why we sweat, what we sweat, and how the toxic stuff that's released through our pores could affect us if we didn't use a sauna. I described in detail the three types of heat conveyance—and how they affect the body differently. (Far infrared is by far the best choice for a sauna, but it has to radiate within a certain bandwidth.) Sauna construction was also discussed, as different materials confer different benefits, some vastly superior to others. An entire chapter was devoted to who may use the sauna and who should not, while another chapter described in great detail how to take a sauna. Finally, I wrote about detoxification programs for getting well and staying well. It was while doing research for this portion of my book that I met Dr. David Root.

David Root, I would find out, was no conventional doctor. The stories he told me about his air combat experiences as an Air Force pilot were certainly exciting, but what really sparked my interest was the research he was doing in the field of sauna therapy. Unlike his colleagues in mainstream medicine, Dr. Root understood that poisons (commonly called "toxins")—both endogenous (from within the body) and exogenous (from the environment, outside the body)— cause cells to malfunction. A cell that is suffocating in waste cannot assimilate and utilize nutrients. It dies, neighboring cells die, and eventually entire organs, glands, and bodily systems malfunction. It's no surprise that a poisoned body is susceptible to all types of infections and degenerative diseases.

Dr. Root shared with me many scientific studies he had co-authored. The language of the titles was typical of what normally appears in medical journals, although the topics were not: "Excretion of a Lipophilic Toxicant Through the Sebaceous Glands: A Case Report"; "Xenobiotic Reduction And Clinical Improvements In Capacitor Workers: A Feasible Method"; "Diagnosis and Treatment of Patients Presenting Subclinical Signs and Symptoms of Exposure to Chemicals with Bioaccumulate in Human Tissue." Behind all that medical terminology, an important message consistently emerged: We humans have a lot of junk in our systems. Most of this junk comes from synthetic chemicals that the human body was never designed to metabolize or neutralize, and usually has a very difficult time removing. These toxins negatively affect us on all levels. They inflame the joints, impede digestion, clog the liver, overwork the heart, and fog the brain. And that's just the beginning of what can go wrong! The articles concluded, unambiguously, that the best way to become healthy is to sweat in a sauna, which will allow the body to eliminate these toxins and function normally.

There was one addition to the body heating program that Dr. Root advocated. Even more effective than sauna therapy was sauna therapy in conjunction with the ingestion of niacin (Vitamin B3). Why was niacin critical? Because many toxins are fat-soluble— meaning that they have an affinity for fat cells, which promptly store them. In the 1960s, a man named L. Ron Hubbard developed a sauna protocol that included niacin because, he discovered, the vitamin has the remarkable ability to pull toxins out of fat cells. Hubbard's purification protocol was implemented in numerous clinics across the United States, and for many years Dr. Root directed the programs.

Most people who have heard of Hubbard know him only as the founder of the Church of Scientology. Dr. Root was quick to point out to me that he was not, and had never been, a Scientologist. However, David Root is a scientist. And, like all true scientists, he is flexible and wise enough to employ effective protocols wherever he finds them. As his clinical trials showed, people became functional and felt better once toxic materials were escorted out of the system, catalyzed by the niacin.

In this Detoxination book, you will learn about toxins, how they can affect you, and how to avoid them. You will learn how and when to take niacin in conjunction with the sauna therapy so the maximum levels of toxins can be mobilized for elimination by the body. And you will be told the precise amounts of additional vitamins, minerals, electrolytes and gut binders to take, so you can stay nutritionally balanced while expelling these poisons. The effects of this cleanse will be permanent, unless you suffer further toxin exposure.

Except for sidebars that quote Dr. Root, this book is written by his son Dan. I had the pleasure to meet Dan fourteen years after my initial contact with his father. It would be difficult to find a more enthusiastic proponent of the Detoxination protocol than Dan. Thanks to his passion for research, his own personal participation in the protocol, and his observation of others who participated, Dan has helped institute major improvements in Hubbard's original design. Now, your sweat session will require only one or two hours a day instead of four or five. Moreover, you will very likely experience a reduction or complete eradication of physical and psychological symptoms—not to mention a renewed sense of well-being—in as few as fourteen days instead of many weeks or months.

How can you utilize this protocol? One way is to become a client at the Roots' Detoxination Wellness Centers, where you will receive medical supervision. It's always a good idea to be monitored if you are prone to seizures or fainting, are very sensitive to high temperatures, or have an especially serious medical condition. However, those who don't require intensive medical supervision (or who cannot travel to one of the Centers) can do this protocol on their own. All over the world, people who have conscientiously followed the Detoxination beta-test program are reporting a cessation of their physical ailments and an improvement in mental clarity. Both inside and outside the Centers, all kinds of health issues are being addressed: arthritis, heart and circulatory problems, digestive impairment, neurological conditions, Lyme and other infections, and even the effects of mold exposure.

As you read this book, please remain open to the many possibilities for your improved health. Even more important, do the protocol. Your willingness to devote a couple of hours every day, over the course of just a few weeks, will yield huge results. Results are not merely subjective. They are backed by extensive medical research, published studies, X-rays, and blood and other laboratory tests. Detoxination works. I think you will be not only pleased, but amazed. I know I was.

Nenah Sylver, PhD

lecturer and consultant in electromedicine and holistic health

author of many articles and books, including

The Holistic Handbook of Sauna Therapy and

The Rife Handbook of Frequency Therapy and Holistic Health, 5th Ed.

www.nenahsylver.com

PREFACE

Around the spring of 2016, the idea to write this book was suggested by our business consultant and dear friend. He overheard a conversation between my father and me about research I'd done on hyperthyroidism and the shocking revelations I'd made.

You see, in 2012 my wife Suzy had her thyroid medically destroyed by Radioactive Iodine (RAI) therapy to treat the condition. We had followed the medical advice of her primary care physician, fully expecting her condition to improve.

When her quality of life worsened, we began to do serious research to understand the underlying cause of her "dis-ease." This journey opened our eyes and changed our perception of conventional medicine forever.

Whether by accident or design[1], people have become dumbed down and lethargic by fluoride, kept moribund by pernicious food

---

[1] https://sustainabledevelopment.un.org/content/documents/Agenda21.pdf

products, and held in perpetual morbidity by noxious substances encountered throughout the day.

Many industries either contribute to the problem or profit from it. Admittedly, our business is one set up to profit from this pervasive issue. We, at least, are transparent about it and give you our solution for the small price of this book!

I wrote this book with the hope that our story can help others, like you, who may be suffering from chronic pain, chronic fatigue, insomnia, obesity, muscle weakness, or other inflammatory conditions. In reality, though, this book is for everyone!

What we learned could have prevented the destruction of Suzy's thyroid and subsequent enslavement to thyroid medication: Toxins and poor nutrition created the underlying causes of her symptoms.

Actually, we found toxins and poor nutrition are at the root of most inflammatory, autoimmune, neurological, and endocrine disorders!

Suzy's maltreated thyroid dis-ease (meaning: opposite of freedom from labor, pain, or physical annoyance; tranquil rest; comfort: to enjoy one's ease) had been reversible without invasive medical procedures! Dealing with the existing buildup of—and continued exposures to—environmental toxins as well as improving our nutritional choices was the *real* solution.

This knowledge sent chills down my spine upon the realization that my father David E. Root, M.D., M.P.H., operates a unique detoxification program, which is designed to remove heavy metals, Persistent Organic Pollutants (POPs) like pesticides, and synthetic chemicals that have accumulated in fat, which could have helped Suzy better than conventional medicine. Unfortunately though, it was too late to help her: the damage to her thyroid gland was done.

Suzy's plight fueled my passion with detoxification and helping others. Unfortunately, toxins and detox are poorly understood by the public. Those who do have awareness of the dangers posed by toxins may seek homeopathic remedies, but nothing else compares to the holistic protocol contained within these pages.

This book is for both the layperson and the healthcare professional alike. We hope it brings better awareness to the problem and provides guidance on the brilliant solution for which my father has become world renowned for pioneering in the field of Occupational Medicine.

Recently the question came up about the meaning of "M.P.H" in my father's title. I believe my friend quipped, "He must be a FAST doctor"!

The "Master of Public Health" degree is an advanced degree few Doctors attempt to achieve. The Master in Public Health professional is versed in clinical practice, in academia-based research, public policy, global health, infectious disease, and much more. Combined with a Preventive Medicine specialty, through additional training, such physicians have become experts in methods for maintaining good health and preventing disease.

These doctors will advise patients on specific diets, exercise regimens, and lifestyle habits that are suited to their particular needs. Preventive Medicine/Wellness Specialists take into account a patient's nutritional deficiencies, physical and cardiovascular capabilities, and daily habits in order to advise specific vitamins and supplements to take, how much physical activity to undertake, and which habits should be broken and replaced with more positive behavior.

Hopefully now you will understand the significance of my father's training and expertise as it applies to sauna detoxification.

Healthcare professionals will find in the Appendix an unpublished 50-page scientific review of the protocol, complete with references, submitted in 1987 to the California Medical Board/Board of Quality Assurance in response to an official investigation of his use of the Hubbard sauna detoxification program. Obviously it was accepted, as he maintains his medical license even into his 80s!

At the end of the book we discuss an exciting opportunity for Naturopathic Doctors, Functional or Integrative Doctors, Chiropractors, Physical Therapists, EMTs, Wellness and Fitness Experts, and others, to become trained and certified in Detoxination. We also encourage you to join the *Detox iNation* Facebook group to keep updated and to participate in the many topical discussions.

This is an interactive book. Links to all the reference sources, forms, calculations, products, and other resources discussed in this book may be easily found at https://www.GetDetoxinated.com/book/.

ACKNOWLEDGEMENTS

I have to start by thanking my wonderful wife, Suzy. Not only is she my inspiration for developing Detoxination, but she has been the most supportive person a husband could want. I wish we could turn back time to before we agreed to "treat" her hypothyroidism with invasive radioactive iodine therapy, for it is now too late to improve her condition with this protocol.

To my parents, I thank you for all your faith in me and the unconditional love you have given me. This book wouldn't exist without my father's initial quest to help two severely ill painters by risking his medical career with an unconventional sauna therapy.

I wish to also thank my brother David E. Root, Jr for his support during the roll out of Detoxination Wellness Centers (DWC).

Special thanks go out to Lou and Stephanie Dedier. Lou originally suggested that I write this book. His personal gym, which was next to our clinic, became the proving ground for our concept. Once he moved on to build his Mimosa House restaurant chain, we developed DWC in Lou's renovated office space.

Suzy and I are fortunate to have dear friends like Lisa and Keith Johnson, who have provided needed sales and marketing advice, plenty of constructive criticism, many hours of brainstorming sessions, and their physical bodies as test subjects. Suzy, Lisa, and our mutual friend Kelly Hunter helped to establish a modified protocol for those afflicted with adrenal fatigue syndrome. We are very grateful for their involvement in the development and growth of the business.

Many thanks go out to our medical and support staff at Sacramento Medical Group, that provides needed medical supervision for our patients undergoing the full 30-day program.

A recent addition to our team, Victoria Kosha, has provided needed formatting of content and tables included in this book. Her outstanding job of representing the 50-page response letter submitted by my father to the California Medical Board (found in the Appendix) far exceeded my expectations.

Illustrations created by Fiverr freelance designer 'Adotstudio' and author photography on the back cover was produced by Kim Oliver of Oliver's Captured Moments.

Finally, my heartfelt thanks go to my editor Nenah Sylver, PhD who has authored *The Holistic Handbook of Sauna Therapy* and *The Rife Handbook of Frequency Therapy and Holistic Health 5th Edition: an integrated approach for cancer and other diseases.* Dr. Sylver, whose grasp of holistic health and sauna therapies, as well as being a writer and educator, has been exceptional for a new author like me to have as his editor.

INTRODUCTION

Whether you came in contact with them by accident, by choice, at work or at home, toxins are omnipresent and they're deteriorating your health slowly and silently.

Dis-ease and cancer rates have exploded with industrialization, yet we're conditioned to accept failing health as a natural function of aging or genetic mutations. This same "social allopathic conditioning" discourages natural remedies in favor of costly medical treatments to mask symptoms, rather than addressing their root causes.

In this book, I'm going to show you how to reverse the damage toxins inflict on your body, mind, and bank account. The program we offer is not taught in medical schools. It should be, though, as it is safer, broader in scope, and more effective than the only therapy offered by conventional medicine, I.V. chelation. This program is based on peer-reviewed, medical research partially conducted by my father in the late 1980s and more than 35 years clinical experience.

Since 1982, my father has personally treated over 4,000 patients who suffered toxic chemical exposures either at their workplace or from natural disasters. He is recognized as the world's leading expert in sauna detoxification, and he has spent many years consulting with international government representatives, supervising detox projects both here and abroad, as well as giving lectures at international medical conferences. Most recently, he appeared in the docuseries *The Real Skinny On Fat* hosted by Montel Williams and Naomi Whittel.

I have been involved with his medical practice, Sacramento Medical Group, since 1985 and have personally undergone this detoxification program several times throughout the years in order to maintain my excellent health. Together we have made program advancements in delivery and effectiveness by harnessing new research and technology, and we now offer this as a preventive/wellness program.

We branded our outpatient protocol *Detoxination*® – the process of removing toxins from the human body. The term *detoxification* connotes rehabilitation from drugs and alcohol, and fails to capture the essence of our life changing program.

Although originally designed for drug addiction rehabilitation and then applied to workplace chemical and radiation exposure injuries, we now recommend this protocol to virtually everybody. Whether you're sick or healthy, Detoxination can improve your quality of life and health.

As the Senior Detoxinician, I now administer the updated protocol in our Centers, provide training to medical professionals, and coach individuals who wish to **Get Detoxinated!**™ in the comfort of their own home.

This book will give you the necessary education and confidence to attempt Detoxination yourself. However, we strongly recommend you work with seasoned Detoxinicians such as ourselves in order to realize the highest gains while reducing potential health risks.

If you're asking yourself why we believe almost everyone needs Detoxination, here are some subjective benefits of Detoxination that have been reported by past clients and patients:

- Feel Better, Renewed
- Improved Overall Health
- Greater Energy
- Raised Cognition & I.Q.
- More Restful Sleep
- Increased Weight Loss
- Reduced Aches and Pains
- Peace of Mind
- Better Skin and Body Scent
- Heightened Sense Perception
- Happier Attitude
- Enhanced Physique, Stamina

Additionally, objective results include lowered blood pressure and cholesterol, and many diabetics have actually reduced or eliminated their diabetes medication upon completion.

Pretty exciting, wouldn't you say?!

This is just a sampling of the many short- and long-term benefits one can achieve from Detoxination. How we accomplish all this will become more obvious, so *read on!*

CHAPTER 1:
Whoever Controls Your Health
Controls Your Wealth

In 2018, the total health care costs for a typical American family of four averaged $28,166, which is up over $3,000 from 2016. This is according to a recent report in US Today[2] which based the estimate on the average cost of health insurance paid by employers and employees, as well as deductibles and out-of-pocket expenses. The same report points out that most employees give little thought to their employer's share of the cost, and only see what appears on their paycheck.

Yet part of their total compensation includes providing these health benefits, which is no different to an employer than wages, payroll taxes, and other employments costs. It gets lost on people that one of the reasons that workers have seen smaller raises is because a large share of the total compensation goes toward higher costs of these

---

[2] Boulton, Guy. "You'll Be Shocked at How Much Health Insurance Costs for a Family of Four." USA Today. June 07, 2018.
https://www.usatoday.com/story/money/business/2018/06/06/health-care-costs-price-family-four/676046002/.

benefits. Benefits which we hope we never need, but when we do need them, we unquestionably turn to conventional medicine.

But while the healthcare industry has produced many lifesaving procedures, devices, tests and drugs, it comes at a high price. Fixing a broken leg, for example, can cost up to $7,000. A 3-day hospital stay, on average, can easily rack up $30,000. Without medical insurance, most of us would be financially devastated by these mostly unplanned events.

Then there are the additional expenses from follow-up visits, physical therapy, and the most costly of them all, medications.

The U.S. pharmaceutical industry in 2016 was valued at 446 billion U.S. dollars, and controlled over 45 percent of the global pharmaceutical market. In 2008 over 3.9 billion prescriptions were written, which averages 14 per American.

In case you're wondering what those 14 prescriptions might cost (not including refills), students at the Virginia Commonwealth University were challenged by their professor to calculate the average cost of a prescription based on data available from the 2012 Medical Expenditure Panel Survey conducted by the U.S. Department of Health & Human Services. The results of their calculations put the average price for a prescription filled in the U.S. in 2012 for civilian, non-institutionalized patients around $92.[3] So the average American may spend $1,288 on their 14 prescription medications.

Health care costs are so astronomically high that many are just one medical emergency away from bankruptcy. In 2005, Harvard

---

[3] Carroll, Norman V. "What's the Average Price of a Prescription?" *Pharmacy Business and Economics* (blog). September 19, 2015.
https://wp.vcu.edu/nvcarroll/2015/09/15/whats-the-average-price-of-a-prescription/.

University researchers found half of all bankruptcies in the U.S. stem from a medical crisis—and the group hardest hit is the middle class.

It is estimated that 2 million households are driven into bankruptcy each year by medical crises, yet three-quarters have health insurance at the onset of their illness. More than half are homeowners, and 50 percent of these households include a member with a college education.

A family of four, for example, spends about $1,300 a month in premiums. The deductible for those plans is $13,000 per year. So once you pay $28,600 out-of-pocket each year, your insurance kicks in. At least you *hope* your insurance kicks in.

Take the case of Maggie Ethridge, writer for The Guardian, who was diagnosed with stage 4 endometriosis and driven to bankruptcy after accumulating over $70,000 in medical copayment bills. Although she and her husband lived debt free, paid into health insurance, and had good incomes, her condition wiped them out. Why? Because the insurance company continually denied to pay for her MRI scans, CT scans, and specialists.

While fighting a severe prognosis, Maggie was also forced to fight her insurance carrier. She used up all her Personal Time Off benefits, destroyed her credit, and had to rely on others. Her story is not uncommon in America.

Financial toxicity, coined by Molly McDonald of The Pink Fund, can impact a patient's ability to complete treatment and contributes to early mortality. "Think about it: People without resources will skip treatments or oral medications to save on co-pays."

By 2013, unpaid medical bills became the #1 cause of bankruptcies.

Then there are ongoing medical concerns, like prescriptions. Many of these drugs are refilled without a second thought as to continued necessity; therefore, some people wind up taking many medications they no longer need. Unfortunately, the consequences of combining pharmaceuticals can be extremely toxic to the body.

> **Dr. Root:** *Patients, and indeed all of us, are exposed to low levels of many different toxic compounds on a daily basis. Even with known drug interactions, the physician, nevertheless, has a difficult time keeping track of the interactions of the many different medications he may prescribe to a single individual. The literature of pharmacology and toxicology is replete with examples in which one agent enhances the effects of others, either directly or indirectly. Reiter notes, "Although one might prefer to know more about the potential effects of toxicants when administered alone before we tackle the problem of mixtures, the 'real world' situation demands the development of a strategy for the evaluation of mixtures."[4]*

It has been estimated that two million people are victims of prescription drug induced illnesses, according to the New England Journal of Medicine.[5] Drug toxicity is linked to obesity, diabetes, cancer, kidney disease, autism, depression, and heart failure in patients.

---

[4] "Diagnosis and Treatment of Patients Presenting Subclinical Signs and Symptoms of Exposure to Chemicals with Bioaccumulate in Human Tissue", David E. Root, David B. Katzin , Ph. D, David W. Schnare, Ph. D, presented – National Conference on Hazardous Wastes and Environmental Emergencies and sponsored by Hazardous Materials Control Research Institute and the U.S. Environmental Protection Agency, May 1985. Cincinnati, OH. https://www.getdetoxinated.com/docs/epa_speech.pdf
[5] "How the AMA Hooks You on Drugs, Harms Your Health and Hurts the Earth." *The People's Chemist* (blog). May 11, 2011. https://thepeopleschemist.com/how-the-ama-hooks-you-on-drugs-harms-your-health-and-hurts-the-earth/.

Medical tests are also potentially hazardous to the health of patients. Take the case of the popular MRI scan, for example.

MRI – Magnetic Resonance Insanity: Toxic Gadolinium

"My highest priority is daily pain and the twisting/squeezing tightness of craniofacial tendons and ligaments. The skin on my scalp feels like an open, gaping wound at the slightest touch. The neuropathy and not having a sense of where my arms and hands are, is just as painful."

These horrific statements are from a respondent to a survey[6] conducted by The Lighthouse Project in 2014 of patients that underwent anywhere from 1 to 8 Magnetic Resonance Imaging tests using a now-controversial intravenous Gadolinium-Based Contrast Agent (GBCA) to enhance images of abnormal tissue.

Gadolinium is extremely toxic to the system in its native state. It must be bound to an organic *chelating agent* (a chemical compound that reacts with metal ions to form a stable, less toxic complex) in order to be administered into the body.

GBCAs are generally thought to be safe to use; however, retention of gadolinium in fat, bone, and brain tissue is known to have serious consequences. Researchers have estimated that approximately 1% (15 mg) of the 1.5 grams of injected gadolinium from each dose of contrast (0.1 mmol/kg body weight) may be dechelated (released) from the contrast agent and deposited in the bones of GBCA exposed patients including those with normal kidney function.[6]

---

[6] Williams, Sharon, and Hubbs Grimm. "Gadolinium Toxicity, A Survey of the Chronic Effects of Retained Gadolinium from Contrast MRIs Plus Updated Gadolinium Retention Information"(pdf). 2014.
https://gdtoxicity.files.wordpress.com/2014/09/gd-symptom-survey.pdf.

Gadolinium is neurotoxic. It inhibits mitochondrial function and induces oxidative stress. The blood-brain barrier is easily disrupted, and this is why gadolinium is deposited in brain tumors and brain lesions such as those seen in Multiple Sclerosis.

Symptoms of having gadolinium poisoning include:

- Deep bone pain, especially arms and legs
- Muscle twitching and weakness
- Itchy skin or thickening of the skin
- Cognitive symptoms and brain fog
- Vision problems
- Tinnitus or ringing in the ears
- Balance problems
- Swelling of extremities
- Hair loss
- Nephrogenic Systemic Fibrosis

Of the 17 patients cited in the study, "pain" was identified as a chronic symptom, along with burning, numbness, tingling, or prickling sensations (aka paresthesia). Also identified by 10 patients were "deep bone pain" and "electric-like feelings."

This study indicates that gadolinium, a highly toxic heavy metal, can be retained in tissues for 79 months (6.5 years) or more. Patients who underwent multiple MRIs are at even greater risk of bioaccumulating gadolinium, even with normal functioning kidneys.

Unfortunately, the onset of their symptoms may take weeks to appear, so the MRI connection isn't immediately apparent. In the study, 100% of the patients experienced symptoms within the first month following contrast MRI, and 59% reported their symptoms almost immediately.

Ninety percent of gadolinium, according to the experts, safely passes through the body in 24 hours after injection [7]; however, heavy metal tests weeks after injection tell a different tale. Take the case of a 6 year-old that I heard about in a social media group, for example, with gadolinium levels of 178.265mcg/g creat. two months after an MRI. The reference range is 0.3 which makes this child's toxicity 600 times the limit! Gadolinium contrast agents have been used in hundreds of thousands of patients over the past couple decades. [8]

There have been many class-action lawsuits filed since 2016 to stop the "insanity" of gadolinium use, since MRIs and MRAs (magnetic resonance angiography) can be performed without this toxic element. The US Food and Drug Administration (FDA) announced in May, 2018, that it would require additional warnings for GBCAs alerting patients to a potential risk of gadolinium retention. However, most patients are unlikely to heed these warnings, and will blindly accept the advice of the medical professionals. Sadly, there are no immediate plans to discontinue gadolinium use.

Tragically, with the most expensive health care system in the world, the United States ranks 12th among the top 13 high-income countries in the ill health of its citizens. [9]

Poor life choices, as a result of ignorance, misinformation, peer pressure, or conscious decision, have led many individuals to

---

[7] Ferris, Nick, and Stacy Goergen. "Gadolinium Contrast Medium (MRI Contrast Agents)." InsideRadiology. Last modified July 26, 2017. https://www.insideradiology.com.au/gadolinium-contrast-medium/.

[8] Fornell, Dave. "The Debate Over Gadolinium MRI Contrast Toxicity." Imaging Technology News. Last modified February 16, 2018. https://www.itnonline.com/article/debate-over-gadolinium-mri-contrast-toxicity.

[9] Etehad, Melissa, and Kyle Kim. "The U.S. Spends More on Healthcare than Any Other Country - but Not with Better Health Outcomes." Los Angeles Times. July 18, 2017. http://www.latimes.com/nation/la-na-healthcare-comparison-20170715-htmlstory.html.

debilitating conditions requiring assistance from family members or outside caregivers. In hindsight, many of these conditions were preventable; nonetheless, these loved ones have become a financial burden.

According to AARP, family caregivers who leave the workforce to care for a parent or loved one lose, on average, nearly $304,000 in wages and benefits over their lifetime. Added to this figure are the additional out-of-pocket costs associated with long term care.

Better Living Through Chemistry

DuPont's famous slogan from 1935 couldn't be further from the truth. Our metabolisms were designed to process out most toxins found in nature, such as the poison or venom of plant and animal life. However, over the course of the last two centuries we have been subjected to *xenobiotics* such as synthetic chemicals, heavy metals, and Persistent Organic Pollutants (POPs) including pesticides, which are overwhelming our natural detoxification systems.

POPs are so damaging that they deserve further discussion. POPs are defined as, "Organic compounds that are resistant to environmental degradation through chemical, biological, and photolytic processes." This resistance to breakdown results in their bioaccumulation in human and animal food chains. These are the pesticides, solvents, industrial chemicals, plasticizers that characterize modern living.

Water Soluble vs. Fat Soluble

Toxins may be classified as either water soluble or fat soluble. Toxins can also be categorized as endogenous (wastes produced by the body) and exogenous (foreign chemicals such as xenobiotics) substances. Water soluble toxins are readily handled by your liver, kidneys, lungs, lymph, colon, and skin. Fat soluble toxins aren't so easily processed because they are *lipophilic,* or fat loving, and dissolve better in oil based things like fat.

Endogenous toxic waste includes free radicals produced by oxidation. While oxygen is needed to support life, high concentrations of it are corrosive and toxic. By combining digested food with oxygen, the body obtains needed energy. However, this metabolic process also generates dangerous free radicals as byproducts. Free radicals are electronically unstable atoms or molecules that are capable of stripping electrons from any other molecules they touch while attempting to achieve stability. In a domino-like chain reaction, these free radicals create more unstable molecules in their wake.

The term "oxidative stress," therefore, is essentially an imbalance between the production of free radicals and the ability of the body to counteract or detoxify their harmful effects through neutralization by antioxidants. Environmental factors, such as natural and artificial radiation, toxins in air, food, water, and tobacco smoke, compound oxidative stress. Oxidative stress is involved in several age-related conditions, including cardiovascular diseases, chronic obstructive pulmonary disease, chronic kidney disease, neurodegenerative diseases and cancer.

Although free radicals do serve the immune system to locate damaged tissue for removal, the damage *they* cause is frequently linked to fatigue, heart disease, premature aging, and reduced liver detoxification. With this understanding of oxidative stress and free radicals, we can better understand their impact on natural detoxification.

The natural detoxification system consists of three phases that process both endogenous and exogenous toxins for excretion from the body. The Phase I detoxification pathway is responsible for breaking down fat soluble toxins and then sending the metabolites to the Phase II detoxification pathways. In Phase II, new substances are built from the metabolites by adding molecules to them, which is called conjugation.

The purpose of the addition or conjugation of new substances to the Phase I toxic metabolites is to convert them into water soluble forms and make them easier to transport, more stable (less toxic) and more functional for the body to excrete.

There are six Phase II detoxification pathways in the body. Each conjugation pathway serves a specific purpose of detoxifying certain toxins and requires specific nutrients to function. These six detoxification pathways include:

- Glutathione conjugation
- Methylation (more on this and the MTHFR gene mutation in the FAQs section beginning on page 149)
- Sulfation
- Acylation/Glycation
- Acetylation
- Glucuronidation

Once the toxic metabolites are conjugated by Phase II enzymes, Phase III molecules transport the stable toxins out of the body through the urine and/or bile.

If your digestive system is unhealthy, your lymphatic system is congested, or the xenobiotic substance is too complex, toxins cannot be processed effectively. When toxin levels get too high overactivity of the Phase I liver detoxification can cause dangerously high levels of free radicals that must be further metabolized by Phase II to protect against cell damage.

Your liver then becomes overwhelmed and less effective, so the unbound lipophilic toxins are sent back out into the bloodstream where they bind with lipid-rich tissues in various parts of your body.

That's right: the toxins that escape the detoxification pathways accumulate in your fat!

Research has proven that xenobiotics can build up in your body, bypass your liver processing, and become stored in your body fat tissues.[10] The brain, breast, and adrenal glands are organs with higher levels of fatty tissue, making these favorite places for toxin stores. Unfortunately, this can cause brain toxicity and hormonal imbalances, leading to damaging side effects like cognitive issues, and fatigue, as well as contributing to infertility and even the development of some forms of cancer.

During a 1987 field study conducted in Semič, Slovenia, while treating PCB contamination in capacitor workers, my father found PCB toxicity to be 200 to 500 times greater in their fat tissues than was detected in blood serum tests. The implications of this revelation were staggering: blood serum tests merely indicated a tiny fraction of the actual toxic "body burden" (the total amount of chemicals in the body). He and his colleagues published several peer-reviewed papers[11, 12] on this finding, which have been cited in over 25 other research papers and books over the following decades.

---

[10] "National Human Adipose Tissue Survey (Nhats) | Risk Assessment Portal | US EPA." U.S EPA Web Server.
https://cfpub.epa.gov/ncea/risk/recordisplay.cfm?deid=55204.
[11] Tretjak, Z., D.E. Root, A. Tretjak, R. Slivnik, E. Edmondson, R. Graves, and S.L. Beckmann. "Xenobiotic reduction and clinical improvements in capacitor workers: A feasible method." *Journal of Environmental Science and Health . Part A: Environmental Science and Engineering and Toxicology* 25, no. 7 (1990), 731-751. doi:10.1080/10934529009375594.

Since cellular membranes are primarily lipid based substances, they present little barrier to lipid soluble compounds, which can freely pass through them. Potentially damaging fat soluble toxins can, therefore, gain free access to cellular interiors, and are much more difficult to remove. Some of these lipophilic substances, like POPs, can remain in fat for more than 30 years.[13]

Heavy metals like aluminum, lead, and mercury, tend to accumulate in the brain. The brain is 60-70% fat, and the blood–brain barrier is incapable of preventing access to these harmful materials. Neurodegenerative disorders, like Alzheimer's disease, Parkinson's, and Autism Spectrum Disorders are linked to accumulations of these heavy metals in the brain.[14, 15]

The body burden of lipophilic xenobiotics is now proven[16] to be a leading cause for most chronic diseases, chronic pain and fatigue,

---

[12] Tretjak, Ziga, Megan Shields, and Shelley L. Beckmann. "PCB Reduction and Clinical Improvement by Detoxification: an Unexploited Approach?" *Human & Experimental Toxicology* 9, no. 4 (1990), 235-244.
https://www.ncbi.nlm.nih.gov/pubmed/2143911.

[13] Zeliger, Harold I. "Exposure to lipophilic chemicals as a cause of neurological impairments, neurodevelopmental disorders and neurodegenerative diseases." *Interdisciplinary Toxicology* 6, no. 3 (2013), 103-110.
https://www.ncbi.nlm.nih.gov/pmc/articles/PMC3967436/.

[14] Strunecka A, Blaylock RL, Patocka J, Strunecky O. Immunoexcitotoxicity as the central mechanism of etiopathology and treatment of autism spectrum disorders: A possible role of fluoride and aluminum. *Surg Neurol Int*. 2018;9:74. Published 2018 Apr 9. https://www.ncbi.nlm.nih.gov/pmc/articles/PMC5909100/.

[15] Kawahara M, Kato-Negishi M. Link between Aluminum and the Pathogenesis of Alzheimer's Disease: The Integration of the Aluminum and Amyloid Cascade Hypotheses. *Int J Alzheimers Dis*. 2011;2011:276393. Published 2011 Mar 8.
https://www.ncbi.nlm.nih.gov/pmc/articles/PMC3056430/.

[16] Schauss, M. (2018). Toxicity and Chronic Illness - The Weston A. Price Foundation. [online] The Weston A. Price Foundation. https://www.westonaprice.org/health-topics/environmental-toxins/toxicity-and-chronic-illness/.

degenerative disorders, and even cancers. The diabetes epidemic is directly correlated with the increased use of POPs in agriculture.[17]

Over-Exposed

Since 1965, over 4 million chemical compounds have been reported in the literature and nearly 1,000 new chemicals are added to the list on an annual basis. As of 2016, the EPA has had more than 87,000 chemicals listed[18] on its inventory of substances that fall under the Toxic Substances Control Act (TSCA). But the agency is struggling to get a handle on which of those chemicals are in the marketplace today and how they are actually being used. Alarmingly, less than 10% have been tested for human safety by a third party, so the only safety studies available typically have been funded by the patent-holding chemical companies. Of those biased studies on individual substances, fewer than 1% have been tested in combinations to observe negative chemical reactions.

Many, if not most, of these chemicals were not naturally occurring. As such, our bodies have not previously been exposed to them, and therefore have not been able to produce metabolic pathways for removing these xenobiotics. To make matters worse, many of these chemicals have very long biologic half-lives and do not clear from the body rapidly. Some toxicants have half-lives in the range of 10 to 12 years, such as polychlorinated biphenyls (PCBs).

The half-life of a substance is the amount of time it takes before half of the active elements are either eliminated or broken down by the

---

[17] Is the Diabetes Epidemic Primarily Due to Toxins?. *Integr Med (Encinitas)*. 2016;15(4):8-17. https://www.ncbi.nlm.nih.gov/pmc/articles/PMC4991654/
[18] "Perils of Paradigm: Complexity, Policy Design, and the Endocrine Disruptor Screening Program." Environmental Health. https://ehjournal.biomedcentral.com/articles/10.1186/1476-069X-4-2.

body. This is repeated for the next half-life duration, and continues on and on for decades.

Historically, chemical manufacturers were only required to take corrective action once an environmental issue or medical concern reached socially unacceptable levels. Fortunately, legislation is being promoted to force chemical companies to prove human safety prior to public release of their products.

In the meantime, we are bombarded by hazardous substances in the air, food, water, textiles, cosmetics, flooring, furniture, and pharmaceuticals we encounter daily. In addition to flame retardants and formaldehyde, heavy metals and petrochemical toxins are the most common and the most detrimental to health.

Petrochemicals are the basis for most common toxins. Plastics, pharmaceuticals, pesticides, air pollution, personal care products, and much more are all petrochemically based.

The EPA reports 3.42 billion chemicals were released to land, water, and air in 2016[19] and world plastics production totaled approximately 738 billion pounds that same year.[20] Plastics usually contain endocrine disrupting chemicals, like Bisphenol A and phthalates which give strength, clarity, and flexibility to the plastics but do so at our expense.

Signaling hormones in the endocrine system control organ formation and growth, sexual maturation, intelligence, mood and bonding behaviors, sleep patterns, appetite and thirst, and stress response.

---

[19] "Releases of Chemicals in the 2016 TRI National Analysis." US EPA. Last modified January 25, 2018. https://www.epa.gov/trinationalanalysis/releases-chemicals-2016-tri-national-analysis.
[20] "Global Plastic Production." Statista. https://www.statista.com/statistics/282732/global-production-of-plastics-since-1950/.

They also influence bone density, blood pressure, blood sugar, cholesterol levels, metabolic level, fat storage, and the ability to fight illness, to name a few.

Endocrine disruptors act by interfering with the biosynthesis, secretion, action, or metabolism of naturally occurring hormones.[21] Petrochemicals, whose origins stem from the extraction, processing, and burning of fossil fuel, are endocrine disruptors. These petroleum distillates are found in perfluorinated compounds, flame retardants, antimicrobials, surfactants, solvents, plastics, and dyes. They are also found in personal care products, household products, cleaning products, electronics furniture, clothing, and children's toys.

BPA was first developed in the 1930s as a synthetic estrogen for hormone replacement drugs, but it failed to live up to expectations. Industry found other uses for BPA, including polycarbonate resins that make up hard plastics, epoxy resins found in the linings of food storage cans and pipes, flame retardants, thermal cash register receipt paper, DVDs, baby bottles, water bottles, eyeglass lenses, cellphones, toys, appliances, sports safety equipment, vehicles, and airplanes.

BPA has been detected in 90% of the people tested.[22] Ingestion from leaching is the primary route of exposure. Leaching occurs when chemical bonds are broken by heat or linings are exposed to pH basic foods or acidic foods like tomatoes.

---

[21] Waring, R.H., and R.M. Harris. 2005. Endocrine disrupters: a human risk? Molecular and Cellular Endocrinology 244 (1-2):2-9. https://www.ncbi.nlm.nih.gov/pubmed/16271281.

[22] Shelnutt, Susan, John Kind, and William Allaben. "Bisphenol A: Update on newly developed data and how they address NTP's 2008 finding of "Some Concern"." *Food and Chemical Toxicology* 57 (2013), 284-295. https://www.sciencedirect.com/science/article/pii/S027869151300210X.

Phthalates, which make plastics softer and more flexible and fragrances last longer, are common in food packaging, where they leach into the products we eat and drink every day. More than 470 million pounds of phthalates are produced or imported in the United States each year

Although used in plastics, phthalates do not bond with the plastic so they readily leach or evaporate off. Phthalates are lipophilic in nature, so contact with fatty foods and oily substances causes leaching from plastic products. These free phthalates are ingested with food products, nutritional supplements, pharmaceuticals, dental sealants, denture materials, medical devices such as fluid bags and tubing, and the mouthing of children's toys.

In 2000 the Centers for Disease Control and Prevention (CDC) measured in humans the presence of metabolites of seven phthalates. Because of the concerns that phthalates interfere with reproduction and may cause cancer a study titled "Levels of Seven Urinary Phthalate Metabolites in a Human Reference Populations" was conducted and later published in the October, 2000, issue of *Environmental Health Perspectives*. Of the seven phthalate metabolites measured in human samples, four were found in more than 75% of the 289 samples analyzed from adults aged 20-60.[23]

Even low concentrations (parts per trillion) cause harm or permanent effects from prenatal and early childhood exposure, and the effects can be expressed over multiple generations. Over 75 human studies showed adverse health effects in the reproductive, thyroid, immune, and metabolic systems.

---

[23] Blount, Benjamin C., Manori J. Silva, Samuel P. Caudill, Larry L. Needham, Jim L. Pirkle, Eric J. Sampson, George W. Lucier, Richard J. Jackson, and John W. Brock. "Levels of Seven Urinary Phthalate Metabolites in a Human Reference Population." *Environmental Health Perspectives* 108, no. 10 (2000), 979. https://www.ncbi.nlm.nih.gov/pmc/articles/PMC1240132/

In utero exposures can lead to spontaneous abortion, childhood obesity, neurodevelopment disruption, behavior issues, and asthma. In children and adults, other effects include increased abdominal obesity and insulin resistance, altered hormone levels, reduced sperm viability, earlier breast development, and asthma. Some of these effects are seen at concentrations 5,000 times lower than government "safe" levels.[24]

The takeaway from this is that low level exposure to endocrine disruptors is harmful, especially for pregnant women and children. These disruptors are found in nearly everything we eat, drink, and touch every day.

You Are What You Consume

Convenience has created a consumer catastrophe. Today it's cheaper, quicker, and deceptively tastier to buy fast food than to run to the supermarket for organic produce and grass-fed meat protein to prepare a home cooked meal. Prepackaged, processed foods contain dyes and phosphate additives that magnify taste, texture, and shelf-life. They may be wrapped in packaging containing phthalates and BPA.

These chemicals may cause rapid aging, kidney failure, and weak bones. Modified foods overstimulate the production of dopamine, leading to salt and sugar cravings while increasing your risk of heart disease, dementia, neurological problems, respiratory failure and cancer.

"Roundup Ready" Genetically Modified Organisms (GMOs) were developed to tolerate massive quantities of the herbicide glyphosate.

---

[24] Rochester, Johanna R. "Bisphenol A and human health: A review of the literature." *Reproductive Toxicology* 42 (2013), 132-155. https://www.healthandenvironment.org/docs/RochesterBPAstudy2013.pdf.

The CDC and USDA have known[25] for years glyphosate is implicated in the increase of many medical conditions, including autism spectrum disorders, celiac disease, diabetes, kidney failure, morbid obesity, cancers, Parkinson's Disease, and Alzheimer's deaths.

A San Francisco jury on August 10th, 2018, found Monsanto, maker of Roundup, liable for a school groundskeeper's non-Hodgkin's lymphoma that he said developed after years of applying the company's popular weed killer.

"The $289-million award in San Francisco County Superior Court is certain to add momentum to a multi-front battle to ban Roundup's main active ingredient, glyphosate. The compound is applied to millions of acres of crops, many of which have been genetically modified to withstand the herbicide," according to the LA Times. [26]

DeWayne Lee Johnson, 46, applied Roundup weed killer 20 to 30 times per year while working as a groundskeeper for a school district near San Francisco, his attorneys said. He testified that during his work, he had two accidents in which he was doused with the product. The first accident happened in 2012.[27]

The California Department of Pesticide Regulation reported that California growers also applied glyphosate to more than 200 crops

---

[25] Swanson, Nancy L., Andre Leu, Jon Abrahamson, and Bradley Wallet. "Genetically Engineered Crops, Glyphosate And The Deterioration Of Health In The United States Of America." *Journal of Organic Systems* 9, no. 2 (September 2014). https://www.organic-systems.org/journal/92/abstracts/Swanson-et-al.html.

[26] Mohan, Geoffrey. "California Jury Awards $289 Million to Man Who Claimed Monsanto's Roundup Pesticide Gave Him Cancer - Los Angeles Times." Latimes.com. Last modified August 11, 2018. http://www.latimes.com/business/la-fi-roundup-verdict-20180810-story.html.

[27] Holly Yan, CNN. "Jurors Give $289 Million to a Man They Say Got Cancer from Monsanto's Roundup Weedkiller." CNN. Last modified August 12, 2018. https://www.cnn.com/2018/08/10/health/monsanto-johnson-trial-verdict/index.html.

across 4 million acres, including 1.5 million acres of almonds, making it their most widely used herbicide.[26]

Although the award was later lowered to an amount around 78 million, this case is just the tip of the iceberg. There are now over 5,000 similar cases filed against Monsanto, a subsidiary of Bayer.

Glyphosate is known to be water soluble, and therefore should not be retained in the body fat. However, in 2013 a research paper was published that revealed a cell vulnerability resulting from lipophilic xenobiotic toxicity. The conclusion to this paper reads:

> The prevalence of neurological diseases, including NIs [Neurological Impairments], NDDs [Neurodevelopmental Disorders] and NDGDs [Neurodegenerative Diseases] is increasing rapidly throughout the world. The evidence presented here strongly suggests that this increase is due in large part to increased exposure to exogenous lipophilic chemicals which, though varying widely in structure, toxicology, chemical reactivity and retention time in the body, render the *body susceptible to attack via subsequent exposure to low levels of hydrophilic toxins that would otherwise not be absorbed.* [Emphasis added] The lipophilic chemicals can be POPs that are metabolized and eliminated slowly, or BPA, phthalates, PAHs [Polynuclear Aromatic Hydrocarbons], LMWHCs [Low Molecular Weight Hydrocarbons] and other lipophilic species that are eliminated from the body more rapidly, but are constantly replenished in the body from polluted air and water and contaminated food. The accumulation of lipophilic chemicals in the body proceeds until a critical lipophilic load level is reached, at which point the body is vulnerable to attack by low levels of toxic hydrophilic chemicals that would otherwise not be toxic.

Sequential absorption of lipophiles followed by hydrophiles provides a unified explanation of how low levels of rather different environmental pollutants are responsible for the alarming increase of neurological diseases.[13]

Glyphosate, too, is an endocrine disruptor as it causes a dangerous iodine deficiency. We discuss the importance of iodine on page 31.

According to MIT research scientist Stephanie Seneff, Glyphosate is possibly *"the most important factor in the development of multiple chronic diseases and conditions that have become prevalent in Westernized Societies."*[28]

Dr. Seneff and Anthony Samsel, a scientist from Deerfield, NH, published a paper linking celiac disease and the growing problem of gluten intolerance to Glyphosate. In this paper, they have systematically shown how all of the features of celiac disease, including gluten intolerance, a higher risk of thyroid disease, kidney disease, cancer, and an increased risk of infertility and birth defects in children born to celiac mothers, can be explained by glyphosate's known properties. These include (1) disrupting the shikimate pathway [used by gut bacteria and plant species for the biosynthesis of folates and aromatic amino acids], (2) altering the balance between pathogens and beneficial biota in the gut, (3) chelating transition metals, as well as sulfur and selenium, and (4) inhibiting cytochrome P450 enzymes.[29]

---

[28] Samsel, Anthony, and Stephanie Seneff. "Glyphosate's Suppression of Cytochrome P450 Enzymes and Amino Acid Biosynthesis by the Gut Microbiome: Pathways to Modern Diseases." *Entropy* 15, no. 12 (2013), 1416-1463. https://www.mdpi.com/1099-4300/15/4/1416.

[29] Samsel A, Seneff S. Glyphosate, pathways to modern diseases II: Celiac sprue and gluten intolerance. *Interdiscip Toxicol*. 2013;6(4):159-84. https://www.ncbi.nlm.nih.gov/pmc/articles/PMC3945755/.

A report found in the *Journal of Organic Systems*[30] presents the correlation curves of most chronic diseases, such as diabetes, kidney failure, autism, Alzheimer's, Parkinson's, obesity, and cancers, to the introduction—and subsequent dominance—of Genetically Modified Organisms or Genetically Engineered (GE) crops, like corn and soy, from 1996 to 2010.

The following graphs are courtesy of Dr. Nancy L. Swanson.

---

[30] "Swanson Et Al - Organic Systems Journal Vol.9 No.2 (2014)." JOS | Journal of Organic Systems. https://www.organic-systems.org/journal/92/abstracts/Swanson-et-al.html.

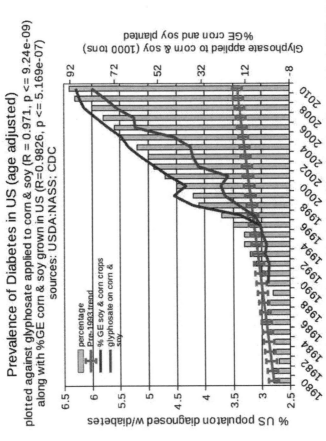

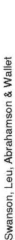

Figure 15. Correlation between age-adjusted diabetes prevalence and glyphosate applications and percentage of US corn and soy crops that are GE.

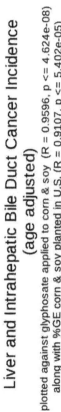
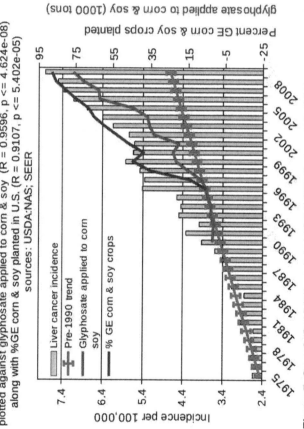

Figure 7. Correlation between age-adjusted liver cancer incidence and glyphosate applications and percentage of US corn and soy crops that are GE.

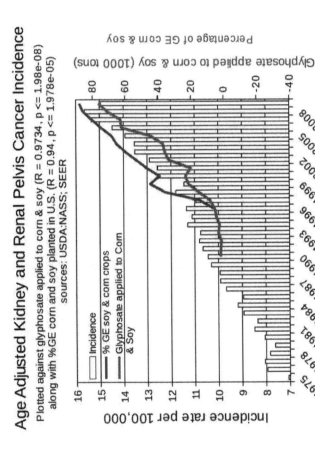

Figure 8. Correlation between age-adjusted kidney cancer incidence and glyphosate applications and percentage of US corn and soy crops that are GE.

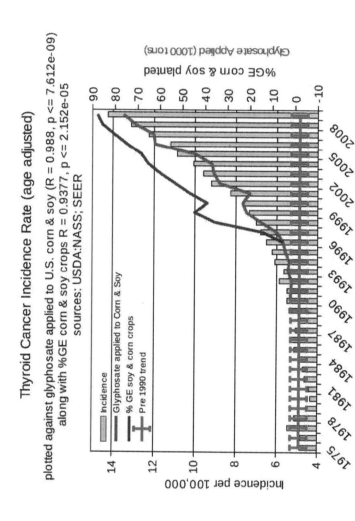

Figure 10. Correlation between age-adjusted thyroid cancer incidence and glyphosate applications and percentage of US corn and soy crops that are GE.

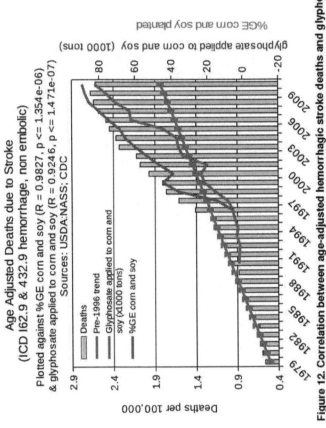

Figure 12. Correlation between age-adjusted hemorrhagic stroke deaths and glyphosate applications and percentage of US corn and soy crops that are GE.

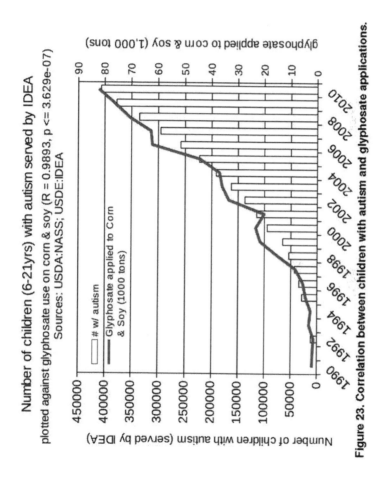

Figure 23. Correlation between children with autism and glyphosate applications.

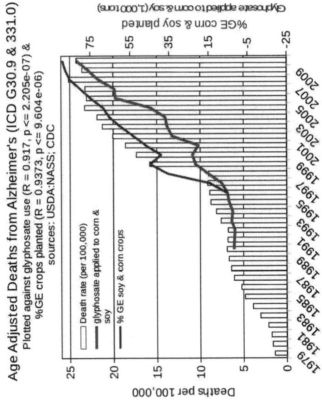

Figure 25. Correlation between age-adjusted Alzheimer's disease deaths and glyphosate applications and percentage of US corn and soy crops that are GE.

Even our municipal water treatment plants are incapable of adequately removing glyphosate and other xenobiotics from the effluent. Globally, over 80 percent[31] of the wastewater generated by society flows back into the ecosystem without being treated.

A frightening example of this problem may surprise you. Many of the chemicals to which we are exposed come from drugs or pharmaceuticals—medications designed for internal use in or on the body. Obviously, medications can be very helpful and indeed lifesaving, but they can also be dangerous if used improperly or by persons who unknowingly drink them in tap water.

The human body will use what it needs of medications and discards the remainder, either partially, completely or not at all, by metabolizing the substances. When these excreted medications reach the sewage treatment plants, much of this material passes through without being removed since these facilities are typically designed to only handle biologic waste, and not chemicals.

Consider that millions of women worldwide take some form of birth control consisting primarily of estrogens and progesterones which pass through the body and end up via the urine in sewage treatment plants. Or when a loved-one passes many times their prescriptions are simply flushed down the toilet by family members tasked with closing the estate. These, too, pass through the plants without being removed or completely neutralized, thereby contaminating people downstream who must use the polluted waters.

In a landmark 1999-2000 USGS survey, 80% of the water samples from 139 American rivers and streams in 30 states were found to be contaminated with drugs, ranging from antibiotics and

---

[31] "Advanced Wastewater Treatment Can Halve Emissions." Baltic Eye. https://balticeye.org/en/pollutants/advanced-wastewater-treatment/.

antidepressants to contraceptives and hormone replacements. Estrogens in the drinking water are linked with testicular cancer, infertility, and childhood "Gender Dysphoria."[32]

Fluoride Fallacy

Today, 74.4% of our water is fluoridated[32] with a compound known as hydrofluorosilicic acid (HFSA). HFSA is a waste byproduct of the aluminum smelting industry, the nuclear industry, and the process used to manufacture phosphate fertilizers.

HFSA, high in arsenic and previously considered to be toxic waste, was illegally dumped into rivers and the environment, but it is now more than likely an additive in your family's water based on junk science and corporate lobbyists. In an unparalleled turn of events, industry shifted the high cost of fluoride disposal into a profit center by convincing bureaucrats and the public to add HSFA to the water supply. Essentially, we have become bio-filters for HSFA disposal.

Research showing that fluoride prevents dental caries (tooth decay and cavities) is biased and unsubstantiated. If fluoride does prevent caries, it is only effective when applied topically. Legitimate research[33] proves that fluoride is a neurotoxin and is also linked to the rise in endocrine[34] disorders, including hypothyroidism, hyper-thyroidism, and Hashimoto's thyroiditis.

Fluoride is the only "drug" added, without our informed consent, to drinking water, and it is impossible to regulate individual doses. If

---

[32] "Is Fluoride Bad for You? Fluoride Facts + Known Dangers." Dr. Axe. Last modified October 15, 2017. https://draxe.com/is-fluoride-bad-for-you/.

[33] "Water Fluoridation: A Critical Review of the Physiological Effects of Ingested Fluoride As a Public Health Intervention." PubMed Central (PMC). https://www.ncbi.nlm.nih.gov/pmc/articles/PMC3956646/.

[34] "The Effects Of Fluoride On The Thyroid Gland." Rense.com. https://rense.com/general57/FLUR.HTM.

toothpaste containing fluoride is swallowed, you *must* call Poison Control to prevent accidental death according to the warning label.

Fluoride is linked to many inflammatory diseases. In large amounts during the first eight years of life, fluoride intake can lead to a permanent mottling of teeth called dental fluorosis.

A major concern is the buildup of fluoride in bone, teeth, and the brain. Of all the structures in your brain, it is the pineal gland that suffers the most.

The pineal gland synthesizes and secretes melatonin, which is essential for your sleep cycle, overnight restoration, and cancer fighting. Fluoride calcification of the pineal gland[35] causes insomnia or sleeplessness, reduced cognitive function and I.Q., lowered immunity, and the dreaded "brain fog."

Another huge health concern with fluoride is the endocrine disrupting nature of this highly reactive element in connection to the thyroid gland and the uptake of iodine.

A great book to read to learn more about the history and dangers of fluoride is called *The Fluoride Deception* by Christopher Bryson.

Importance of Iodine

Iodine is an important trace element needed by every cell in the body, and it is essential for thyroid health. Iodine is the base molecule of thyroid hormone and the thyroid needs iodine to produce it. Iodine deficiency is a major cause of cystic diseases, including goiters (thyroid cysts), fibrocystic breast disease,

---

[35] Kunz D, et al. (1999). A new concept for melatonin deficit: on pineal calcification and melatonin excretion. Neuropsychopharmacology 21(6):765-72. https://fluoridealert.org/issues/health/pineal-gland/.

fibromyalgia, and uterine fibroids (endometrial polyps and ovarian cysts).

Iodine deficiencies are also notable with symptoms of:

- Brain fog
- Depression
- Insomnia
- Dry skin
- Hair loss
- Afternoon fatigue and/or weakness
- Cold hands, feet, and low body temperature
- Tongue feeling enlarged
- Immune system problems (always sick)
- Slow metabolism and trouble losing weight

The National Health and Nutrition Survey from 1971 to 2000 showed iodine levels had dropped 50 percent from 1971 to the year 2000.[36] This alarming trend is linked to the increased diagnoses of hypothyroidism. Iodine deficiency has been directly associated with miscarriages, stillbirth, pre-term delivery, and cognitive problems (low I.Q. and mental retardation).[37] Expecting mothers need 2-3 times the amount of iodine during pregnancy.

Over 20 million Americans have some form of thyroid disease, and one in eight women will develop a thyroid disorder during her lifetime.[37] In the U.S. 13 of the top 50 selling drugs are some form of thyroid hormone. (The fourth highest selling drug is Levothyroxine.) Hypothyroidism, one of the most common thyroid disorders, is an autoimmune disease which is linked to iodine-displacing halogens.

The halogen group of the periodic table includes fluorine, chlorine, bromine, iodine, and astatide (radioactive, rare, and not often found in nature). Of these, iodine is the only halogen required by the body.

---

[36] "Products - Health E Stats - Iodine Levels in the United States, 2000." Centers for Disease Control and Prevention. Last modified February 3, 2010. https://www.cdc.gov/nchs/data/hestat/iodine.htm.

[37] "General Information/Press Room." American Thyroid Association. Accessed December 2, 2018. https://www.thyroid.org/media-main/press-room/.

No one gets enough iodine in their diet unless they take it as a supplement. Fluoride and bromine, used to sanitize hot tubs and in bread and other baked goods as potassium bromate (a bleaching agent), fool iodine receptors in the thyroid. These elements mimic iodine molecules thus preventing the production of thyroid hormone that regulate the body's metabolic rate as well as heart and digestive function, muscle control, brain development, and bone maintenance.

Iodine intake immediately increases the excretion of bromide, fluoride, and some heavy metals including mercury and lead. Dr. Kenezy Gyula Korhaz states that iodine chelates heavy metals such as mercury, lead, cadmium, aluminum and halogens, thus decreasing their iodine inhibiting effects.[38]

The white blood cells of the immune system need iodine to fight infection. Iodine is a great antiseptic. To this day, there's no bacteria, virus, or any other microorganism that can survive or adapt to being in an iodine-rich environment. So it does help to protect your immune system from invading micro-organisms.[39]

We cannot tell you what your recommended daily amount should be; this is something you should have properly tested. We can recommend that you take nascent iodine or Lugol's iodine daily. Avoid iodine tinctures containing alcohol, and seek iodine in a vegetable-glycerin base.

[38] Sticht, G., Käferstein, H., Bromine. In Handbook on Toxicity of Inorganic Compounds – Seiler HG and Sigel, H Editors, Marcel Dekker Inc, 143-151, 1988.
[39] "Everything You Need To Know About Iodine Webinar by Dr. Edward F. Group." *Dr. Group's Healthy Living Articles* (blog). September 7, 2016. https://www.globalhealingcenter.com/natural-health/free-iodine-webinar/.

The following table 1.1 is provided by the National Institutes of Health, Office of Dietary Supplements.[40] The amount of iodine you need each day depends on your age. Average daily recommended amounts are listed below in micrograms (mcg).

Table 1.1

Life Stage	Recommended Amount
Birth to 6 months	110 mcg
Infants 7-12 months	130 mcg
Children 1-8 years	90 mcg
Children 9-13 years	120 mcg
Teens 14-18 years	150 mcg
Adults	150 mcg
Pregnant teens and women	220 mcg
Breastfeeding teens and women	290 mcg

[40] "Office of Dietary Supplements - Iodine." *Office of Dietary Supplements (ODS)* (blog). February 17, 2016. https://ods.od.nih.gov/factsheets/Iodine-Consumer/.

Emerging Concerns

Today, the social media buzz is on infants and excessive vaccine schedules. Given the recent whistle-blower testimonies[41] and third-party research[42] regarding contaminated vaccines and lack of safety studies, this concern is extremely valid. Often overlooked, however, is the real danger your toxic body burden presents to your unborn child. When planning a family, couples need to consider not only their genetic traits, but their xenobiotic transmission to their developing fetus as well. Mothers will pass their chemical contamination through the placenta and umbilical cord during gestation, and then feed their baby toxic breast milk.

Studies[43] have shown that breasts contain the highest concentrations of hazardous substances, such as arsenic, cadmium, lead and aluminum. Even in lower exposures of parts per *trillion*, these xenobiotics can lead to endocrine disruption, immune suppression, birth defects, and reproductive failure.

In 2005, the Environmental Working Group published their report on "The Pollution in Newborns,"[44] where ten randomly selected samples of umbilical cord blood were tested. The EWG study detected 287 chemicals, most of which are toxic to the brain and nervous system. Of these, 208 chemicals are known to cause birth defects, 180 cause

---

[41] "CDC Whistleblower and Corruption." A Voice for Choice.
http://avoiceforchoice.org/cdcwhistleblower/.
[42] McGovern, Celeste. "Dirty Vaccines: New Study Reveals Prevalence of Contaminants." http://info.cmsri.org/the-driven-researcher-blog/dirty-vaccines-new-study-reveals-prevalence-of-contaminants.
[43] "Arsenic, Cadmium, Lead, and Aluminium Concentrations in Human Milk at Early Stages of Lactation." ScienceDirect.com | Science, Health and Medical Journals, Full Text Articles and Books.
https://www.sciencedirect.com/science/article/pii/S1875957213001502.
[44] "Body Burden: The Pollution in Newborns." EWG.
https://www.ewg.org/research/body-burden-pollution-newborns.

cancers in humans or animals, and nine of the cord blood samples tested positive for Bisphenol A (BPA) used in plastics.

Occupational Hazards

Chronic chemical exposures from fume inhalation and skin contact in the workplace is the eighth leading cause of death in the nation.[45]

If you're in the military or industries such as mining, agriculture, chemical production, construction, manufacturing, healthcare, firefighting, transportation, or textiles then you likely have been chronically exposed to toxic substances that deteriorate your health slowly and silently.

It has been reported that 160 million occupational diseases are diagnosed per year. Most of these occupational diseases are caused by chemical agents.[46]

Too often, employers allow hazardous substances to be mishandled, they issue inferior Personal Protective Equipment (PPE), or they provide inadequate safety, storage, and handling instruction. When spills or unintentional exposures occur, the contamination can quickly spread through the air, soil and water, and be absorbed through your skin or lungs, or by ingestion.

Employers often do not disclose these Occupational Safety and Health Administration regulation violations because they'd be heavily fined.

---

[45] "Silent Epidemic Of Workplace Chemical Exposures Rages On." PEER - Home. https://www.peer.org/news/press-releases/silent-epidemic-of-workplace-chemical-exposures-rages-on.html.

[46] "ILO Calls for Urgent Global Action to Fight Occupational Diseases." International Labour Organization. Last modified April 26, 2013. https://www.ilo.org/global/about-the-ilo/newsroom/news/WCMS_211627/lang--en/index.htm.

Corporate Wellness Programs—heralded to be a great solution to the problem of absenteeism due to illness—differ widely across companies, but they all aim to reduce sick days and increase employee productivity. Sadly, these well intentioned programs fail to address the real issue: illness caused by accumulated xenobiotics.

Common workplace toxic exposures include asbestos, benzene, arsenic, ammonia, chloroform, zinc, lead, mercury, iodine, formaldehyde, hydrogen peroxide, uranium, and many more.

Conservative estimates indicate at least 1 in 10 cancers are the result of preventable and predictable workplace exposure. More people face a risk of occupational cancer today than at any other time in history.

The International Labour Organization (ILO) estimates the human toll from occupational cancer at over 609,000 deaths per year—one death every 52 seconds.[47] The estimate from non-governmental sources goes up to 810,000 occupational cancer deaths.[48]

Cancer now ranks as the leading cause of death amongst fire fighters, according to the International Association of Firefighters.[49]

Emergency service professionals are classified by the insurance industry as *high hazard* and demonstrate an alarmingly high incidence of heart attack, high blood pressure, and cancer.

---

[47] Päivi Hämäläinen, Jukka Takala, Kaija Leena Saarela. Global estimates of fatal work-related diseases, American Journal of Industrial Medicine (AJIM), volume 50, pages 28-41, 2007. https://onlinelibrary.wiley.com/doi/abs/10.1002/ajim.20411.

[48] Cancerresearchuk.org estimates 8.1 million cancer deaths/year worldwide (2012). Applying the 1/10 ratio of occupational cancers lead to the 810,000 figure.

[49] "Cancer is the Biggest Killer of America's Firefighters." NBC News. Last modified October 23, 2017. https://www.nbcnews.com/health/cancer/cancer-biggest-killer-america-s-firefighters-n813411.

According to *Firehouse Magazine*, when compared to the general population, firefighters demonstrate[50]:

- 100% higher risk of developing testicular cancer
- 50% higher risk for multiple myeloma, an incurable bone cancer
- 50% higher risk for non-Hodgkin's lymphoma
- 28% higher risk of prostate cancer
- Increases in brain, colon and thyroid cancers and malignant melanoma
- Increases in breast cancer

Even if your employer took all reasonable precautions, this does not eliminate your right to a worker's compensation claim if you were exposed to toxic chemicals at work. Workers' comp recovery is not based on fault. All that is required for a workers' compensation claim is that you were exposed to the dangerous substance in the course of your employment, and that the exposure caused an illness or other bodily harm.

Although a Worker's Compensation claim may be filed, there are only a few types of benefits you may be eligible to receive, according to AllLaw.com:

- Temporary disability benefits to compensate for the loss of income during the period you are receiving treatment and unable to work.
- Permanent partial disability or permanent total disability benefits to compensate for permanent bodily impairment due to the toxic exposure.

---

[50] "Hot Zone Design: Contain the Contaminants." Firehouse. https://www.firehouse.com/stations/building-components/article/11588372/station-design-supplement.

- Coverage of your medical treatment expenses, including diagnostic studies, medication, and equipment.

Notice there's no mention of reducing the body burden of the xenobiotics in order to improve your quality of life or health. You are expected to accept your settlement—and fate.

The Sky Is Falling!

Even more controversial are Geoengineering[51] programs by specially-equipped aerosol spraying airplanes which pollute our air with nanoparticles of aluminum, barium, and strontium. Our bodies absorb these particles through the skin and lungs, and ingest with our food and water. The term "chemtrails" conjures up conspiracy theories and incredulity, but a vapor trail from jet engines lasting longer than three minutes is air pollution containing nanoparticles of aluminum oxide, barium, and other harmful exhaust byproducts.

Between 1988 and 1996, all NATO aircraft switched from gasoline-based fuel (JP-5) to kerosene, a diesel fuel (JP-8). The aluminum and barium emissions have now quadrupled, along with increases in many other toxic chemicals.[52] Flight crews report smelling and tasting JP-8 long after exposures, and many suffer a hearing disorder likened to dyslexia of the ears.[53]

---

[51] Chelsea Harvey,E&E News. "World Needs to Set Rules for Geoengineering Experiments, Experts Say." Scientific American. Last modified May 23, 2018. https://www.scientificamerican.com/article/world-needs-to-set-rules-for-geoengineering-experiments-experts-say/.

[52] Lee, Jim. "Aluminum, Barium, and Chemical Trails Explained ? JUST THE FACTS · ClimateViewer News." *ClimateViewer News* (blog). March 15, 2015. https://climateviewer.com/2015/03/15/aluminum-barium-and-chemical-trails-explained-just-the-facts/.

[53] "Exposure to Jet Fuel, Not Just Noise, Contributes to Hearing Problems." *Office of Research & Development* (blog). March 20, 2014. https://www.research.va.gov/currents/spring2014/spring2014-11.cfm.

According to renowned neurosurgeon Russell Blaylock MD, "nanoparticles of aluminum are not only infinitely more inflammatory, they also easily penetrate the brain by a number of routes, including the blood and olfactory nerves (the smell nerves in the nose). Studies have shown that these particles pass along the olfactory neural tracts, which connect directly to the area of the brain that is not only most effected by Alzheimer's disease, but also the earliest affected in the course of the disease. It also has the highest level of brain aluminum in Alzheimer's cases."

Multiple Chemical Sensitivity (MCS)

When the toxic body burden reaches a certain level (this varies by individual), additional bioaccumulations or casual exposures to chemical smells, tastes, or skin contact can become the "straw that broke the camel's back." These tipping point symptoms can include headache, fatigue, dizziness, nausea, congestion, itching, sneezing, sore throat, chest pain, changes in heart rhythm, breathing problems, muscle pain or stiffness, skin rash, diarrhea, bloating, gas, confusion, trouble concentrating, memory problems, and mood changes.

Possible triggers that set off people's symptoms vary a lot, too. They include tobacco smoke, auto exhaust, perfume, insecticides, new carpet, chlorine, and more. Although these feelings and symptoms are very real, health experts cannot agree that *Multiple Chemical Sensitivity* (MCS) is an illness. Many call it "idiopathic environmental intolerance," but it is also known as "environmental illness" or "sick building syndrome."

> **Dr. Root:** *As an example of the "straw that broke the camel's back" I note a patient who was never treated but illustrates this point very graphically:*

This was a 50-year-old lady who had spent 20 years as an artist, painting oil-based pictures and putting out at least 20 paintings a year over a period of 20 years. She had no problems related to the exposure to these paints or solvents, which she used to clean the brushes and thin the paints. However, on one Fall afternoon, she was on the escalator at Macy's going from the second to the third floor where a Macy's employee was cleaning the brass metal work of the escalator with metal cleaner. As this woman ascended into this cloud of cleaning solvent, she immediately became disoriented, felt faint, and knew that she had to remove herself from the area rapidly, though she did not know what was happening. She went to the nearest elevator and when the door opened, did not have the presence of mind to get out of the way to let the people out of the elevator! She got into the elevator, made her way to the ground floor and once outside, knew she could not drive because she was so affected, but attempted to call her husband on her cell phone. She could not remember her husband's cell phone number because of the disorientation. This case very graphically illustrates the principle that we all have an upper limit of chemical exposure and when that exposure is overwhelming, then the person's neurologic and other systems tend to breakdown. Undoubtedly, her 20 years of frequent exposure to paints and solvents put her in harm's way for the final exposure on the escalator.

In May, 1985, my father presented his report, *Diagnosis and Treatment of Patients Presenting Subclinical Signs and Symptoms in Exposure to Chemicals Which Bioaccumulate in Human Tissue,* to the U.S. Environmental Protection Agency (EPA)—effectively injecting the MCS issue into mainstream medicine discourse.

No Relief

The Mt. Sinai School of Medicine performed a small, but telling, research project[54] with nine volunteers in 2003. Their study found a total of 167 xenobiotics between the study participants, with 94 known to affect the brain and nervous system. Each participant averaged 91 hazardous chemicals, 79 of which were linked to birth defects. Shockingly, 76 chemicals found in all nine subjects were carcinogenic.

There are no acceptable levels of xenobiotics, and to this day conventional medicine has no safe treatment for reducing your body burden of these illness-causing, fat-stored toxins. The only medical therapy specifically for severe heavy metal exposures is chelation.

The I.V. form of chelation involves intravenous injections of one of several chelating chemical agents which binds to heavy metals in blood. Chelating agents can also be administered orally, but either way chelation therapy may remove the good metals with the bad.

If the natural detoxification pathways are impaired, any reduction in good elements, such as iron and copper, can produce unwanted side effects including dehydration, low blood calcium, harm to kidneys, increased enzymes (as would be detected in liver function tests), allergic reactions, and lowered levels of dietary elements. Mobilizing lead without enhancing elimination pathways carries the risk of redistributing lead from bone (its main depot in the body) to soft tissues such as brain and liver, or it could simply redeposit the lead into bone. Similarly, dislodging mercury from tissues may deposit this highly neurotoxic element into the brain tissues.

---

[54] "News - Body Burden: The Pollution in People." Welcome to HeadLice.org. https://www.headlice.org/news/2004/bodyburden.htm.

For people with chronic low-level exposures, as with most of us, chelation therapy is not recommended.

The effects from chemicals that lodge in the body are not always easy to describe. First, there is inadequate health data on the vast majority of the 100,000 chemicals in commercial production. What data does exist tends to reflect effects in rodents rather than humans, and is nearly always the result of large, acute exposures to a single chemical. It is difficult, if not impossible, to estimate the effects of chemical mixtures, and there have been very few such tests in animals. In addition, animal tests are notoriously poor at indicating the potential effects on the skin or the nervous system of humans.

There are also a number of individual and environmental variables which modulate the effects of xenobiotic contamination in humans. Individual variables include:

- Genetic susceptibility or predisposition
- Age
- Nutritional status
- Lifestyle habits, such as alcohol and cigarette consumption
- Biochemical uniqueness as it relates to the efficiency of metabolic pathways for absorption, uptake into tissues and excretion
- The degree of affinity of certain target tissues for xenobiotics in the body
- The presence and degree of psychosocial stresses
- The absence or presence of pre-existing disease.

Environmental variables include:

- Degree of exposure
- Duration of exposure
- The specific chemicals entering the body

- The interactions of chemicals inside the body:
  - o Synergistic (combined effect greater than the sum of the effects of the individual agents);
  - o Potentiating (one component enhancing the effects of another);
  - o Additive (combined effect is the sum of the effects of the individual agents);
  - o Antagonistic (combined effect is less than the sum of the effects of the individual agents).
- The latent period between exposure and effect.

Eminent environmental scientist René Jules Dubos predicted in the 1970s, *"The greatest danger of pollution may well be that we shall tolerate levels of it so low as to have no acute nuisance value, but sufficiently high, nevertheless, to cause delayed pathological effects and despoil the quality of life."*[55]

Joseph Pizzorno, ND, is one of the world's leading authorities on science-based natural/integrative medicine. He is a co-founder of Bastyr University, established in 1978, and the author of *Total Wellness* and co-author of the internationally acclaimed *Textbook of Natural Medicine* and its companion books, *Natural Medicine Instructions for Patients* and the *Handbook of Natural Medicine.* He also co-authored *Encyclopedia of Natural Medicine, Natural Medicine for the Prevention and Treatment of Cancer,* and *Encyclopedia of Healing Foods.* From an editorial piece in the spring, 2013, issue of *Vita Link: The journal of the Canadian Association of Naturopathic Doctors,* Dr. Pizzorno states, "At this time, I estimate that 75% of the general population is suffering some dysfunction and increased risk

---

[55] Rene Dubos, "Adapting to Pollution," Scientist and Citizen 10 (January/February 1968): 1-8.

of serious disease from chemical exposure. This number is, of course, certainly higher in patients suffering chronic disease."[56]

The following table (1.1) from a report presented by my father to the EPA in 1985[57] shows various symptoms associated with six studied chemicals, including Benzene, Disulfide, Dioxin, Lead, PBB, and PCB.

[56] Pizzorno, MD, Joseph. "Persistent Organic Pollutants: A Serious Clinical Concern." Journal of the Canadian Association of Naturopathic Doctors 20, no. 1 (Spring), 11-14. http://www.cand.ca/wp-content/uploads/2016/04/v20_i1_Spring2013_EnviroExposures_LR.pdf.pdf

[57] "Diagnosis and Treatment of Patients Presenting Subclinical Signs and Symptoms of Exposure to Chemicals with Bioaccumulate in Human Tissue", David E. Root, David B. Katzin , Ph. D, David W. Schnare, Ph. D, presented – National Conference on Hazardous Wastes and Environmental Emergencies, May 1985. Cincinnati, OH. http://citeseerx.ist.psu.edu/viewdoc/summary?doi=10.1.1.497.4725.

Table 1.1

SYMPTOM	BENZENE	DISULFIDE	DIOXIN	LEAD	PBB	PCB
Impaired Memory		•		•		•
Confusion		•				
Slowed Adolescent Develop.				•		
Headaches		•		•	•	•
Sleeplessness		•		•	•	•
Sleepiness				•	•	•
Eye Irritation					•	•
Dimness Of Sight			•			
Blurred Vision					•	
Eye Oscillation		•				
Pupil Reactions				•		
Weight Loss > 10 Lbs.					•	•
Nausea					•	•
Vomiting				•		
Abdominal Pain						•
Abdominal Cramps					•	
Diarrhea					•	
Joint Pain					•	•
Swelling Of Joints					•	
Muscular Aches & Pains					•	•
Speech Impairment						•
Muscle Weakness		•		•	•	
Tremors				•		
Difficulty Walking				•		
Seizures				•		
Incoordination				•	•	
Dizziness				•	•	•
Fatigue				•	•	•
Depression		•		•	•	•
Nervousness	•		•	•	•	•
Irritability	•	•	•	•		
Emotional Instability		•		•		
Vision Impairment				•	•	
Hearing Impairment				•		
Loss Of Smell/Hearing					•	
Burning Sensation					•	•
Paresthesias		•		•	•	•
Hallucinations		•				
Rash					•	•
Acne					•	•
Sun Sensitivity					•	
Skin Darkening/Thinckening					•	•
Discolor/Deformity Of Nails				•	•	•
Dryness Of Skin				•	•	
Increased Sweating				•	•	
Slow/Poor Healing Of Cuts				•	•	

Cancer Connection

For generations cancer was believed to be primarily a genetic condition, where one was predisposed to whatever particular cancers plagued their relatives and ancestors. In recent years, however, research has firmly connected most cancers with damage to cell mitochondria from xenobiotics and poor nutrition.

In November of 2017, my father was asked to present his 35 years' experience in sauna detoxification at the Tripping Over The Truth conference in Baltimore, Maryland. This event, which brought together international experts in cancer research, oncology, nutrition and detoxification, was hosted by his friend and colleague, Dr. George Yu. Dr. Yu first learned of my father and his work in 2002 after his presentation on nutrition and terminal cancer patients for the Kushi Institute at the National Cancer Institute.[58]

The goal of the Tripping Over The Truth conference was, as Dr. Yu put it, to "blast the world with a new understanding: the environment of food and nutrition and the mechanisms of metabolism and oxygen are the first factors in the mitochondrial dysfunction that occurs before nuclear DNA becomes unstable, and the two together lead to cancers and degenerative 'diseases.' This is a paradigm shift from Darwinian random Somatic Mutational Theory to Lamarckian environmental and metabolic vectors determining the animal's adaptability in mutations for survival and procreation."[59]

After learning from my father about sauna detoxification, Dr. Yu was spurred on to research *in vivo* (performed or taking place in a living organism) biopsies of patients undergoing elective surgery to measure toxic chemical loads in fatty tissues from all over the body.

---

[58] Yu, MD, George. "Cleanse and Detoxification - Totally Yu!" Home - Totally Yu!. https://totallyyu2.com/cleanse-and-detoxification.html.

[59] From a speakers' informational handout received from the conference hosts.

The findings showed that among the numerous chemicals assayed, DDE (a metabolite of DDT) was in everybody's fat cells at a concentration of over 1,000 times higher than found in blood serum levels.[60] "The trouble is we cannot see it or touch it and we don't fully understand what it is doing to us!" said Dr. Yu.[58]

Dr. Yu, himself, began working with the protocol detailed in this book, and in 2014 he was interviewed about the protocol by Dr. Joseph Mercola (mercola.com).[61]

Both my father and Dr. Yu eventually became advisors for the Heroes Health Fund, dedicated to restoring the quality of life to those who serve, and other organizations that will be discussed later in this book. Through their efforts, Dr. Yu and my father helped promote this protocol, which you will learn about momentarily, into the mainstream.

---

[60] G. W. Yu, J. Laseter, and C. Mylander, "Persistent organic pollutants in serum and several different fat compartments in humans," Journal of Environmental and Public Health, vol. 2011, Article ID 417980, 8 pages, 2011. https://www.hindawi.com/journals/jeph/2011/417980/.

[61] Mercola, D.O., Joseph. "Niacin, Exercise, and Sauna: Detoxification Program for You." Mercola.com (blog). May 4, 2014. https://articles.mercola.com/sites/articles/archive/2014/05/04/detoxification-program.aspx.

Recap

The problem of toxic body burden is deeper than reported—quite literally. Blood tests belie the true extent of bioaccumulated hazards that slowly and silently deteriorate our health. Hazardous substances are pervasive in our daily lives, and we've been conditioned to accept them.

Many of the chemicals that industry has created do not metabolize easily; they were developed so that they would not easily or quickly break down. Once in the blood, these chemicals have the opportunity to reach and affect every part of the body.

Most inflammatory conditions, degenerative disorders, and cancers are caused by xenobiotics and poor nutrition. To this day, mainstream medicine has no *safe* or *effective* way to reduce the body burden of lipophilic xenobiotics.

These are some signs your body is overwhelmed by fat-stored xenobiotics:

- Chronic Pain
- Chronic Fatigue
- Insomnia / Sleeplessness
- Bloating and indigestion
- Headaches
- Joint pain
- Weight gain / Obesity
- Brain fog
- Low Testosterone / E.D.

- Forgetfulness / Memory issues
- Constipation or Diarrhea
- Excess gas and smelly stool
- Sinus congestion
- Heartburn
- Food cravings
- Water retention
- Rashes and other skin disorders
- Puffy, dark circles under eyes

Medical expenses continue to escalate as the physical health of Americans deteriorates. It is time to reverse the damage and take control of your own health—*your greatest wealth!*

CHAPTER 2:
The Solution

"If You Haven't Got Your Health, You Haven't Got Anything" (The Princess Bride)

Since the mid-90s, a cottage industry has developed around the concept of "detoxification," or "detox." Although detoxification has, for many generations, been associated with drug and alcohol rehabilitation, it has nonetheless exploded onto the popular culture scene in the form of juice cleanses, detox diets, ionic foot baths, fasting, and even one-hr sauna detox sessions. Now a multi-billion dollar industry, detoxing is seen as necessary by some and bogus by others.

The *idea* is sound. However, most therapies marketed today serve only to feed corporate greed while providing a modicum of support to the liver, kidneys, and GI tract in converting simple toxins into easily eliminated, water soluble waste. Fat soluble toxins stored in adipose and brain tissues are mostly unaffected by these methods.

Fortunately for all of us, my father's discoveries and research were conducted while validating the only known technique to safely and effectively reduce the body burden of xenobiotics: the Hubbard Sauna Detoxification Method—the basis from which we developed our improved program.

Reduction of fat stored chemicals must be aimed at mobilizing toxins from fat stores, distributing the mobilized toxins to routes of elimination, and increasing the rate at which these routes are utilized. This is the design behind the detoxification procedure developed by L. Ron Hubbard in the 1970s.

Originally conceived to combat the threat of radiation contamination from atomic bomb testing in the 50s, Hubbard later refocused his program development to reduce the levels of drug residues in recovering addicts. *Narconon International*, a substance abuse treatment program, has been successfully using the Hubbard Detoxification Method since the 1970s.[62]

Under conditions of heat, exercise or even stress, remnants of drugs can be released from the energy-producing fat cells during *lipolysis* (explained next) then these drug residues bind with receptors in the brain triggering intense cravings. Many poor souls have lost their battle to addiction because these lipophilic chemicals were never properly handled. This may be a major factor in the shockingly high relapse rate of 85%[63] in the drug addiction treatment industry.

Understanding Lipolysis

Your body produces energy during periods of fasting, exercise, or other strenuous activities by breaking down the triglycerides from

---

[62] While Hubbard and Narconon International are connected with the Church of Scientology, we are not. My father was for many years the Chief of the Scientific Advisory Board of Narconon International. He has not been active in that capacity for many years.

[63] Sinha R. New findings on biological factors predicting addiction relapse vulnerability. *Curr Psychiatry Rep.* 2011;13(5):398-405.

fat reservoirs in fat cells into more useable forms, in a process called *lipolysis.*

In order to explain lipolysis, we must first examine the makeup of a fat cell. Fat cells, also called *adipocytes,* make up the adipose tissue we call body fat. Although there are white fat cells, brown fat cells, and marrow fat cells, we are only concerned with white fat cells in this book.

Fat cells contain structures common to most other cells—such as a nucleus (that contains the majority of the cell's genetic material organized as DNA molecules) and mitochondria (which produce energy and regulate cell metabolism)—but these fat cells also contain a reservoir of fat (lipids) surrounded by a layer of cytoplasm.

Each fat reservoir contains a large lipid droplet made up of many molecules of triglycerides and cholesteryl ester. Due to the lipophilic nature of certain toxins, they also accumulate in the fat reservoir.

The following illustration (Figure 2.1) depicts a fat cell containing lipophilic toxins. Note that the cell membrane width has been exaggerated in order to emphasize the *lipid bilayer* (a thin polar membrane made of two layers of lipid molecules. These membranes are flat sheets that form a continuous barrier around all cells.) and *channel proteins* (proteins that allow the transport of specific substances across a cell membrane).

Fig. 2.1

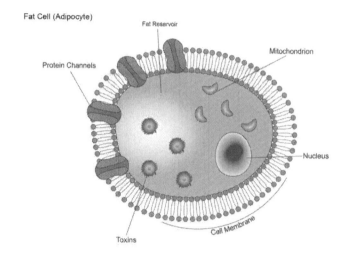

Lipolysis, as shown in Figure 2.2, breaks the chemical bonds of triglycerides, splitting them into their simple components of glycerol and fatty acids. Once fatty acids bind with plasma proteins called albumin and are released from the fat cell, your body uses these Free Fatty Acids (FFAs) to fuel body movement, create heat, and provide energy for body processes.

Before the FFAs are able to be transported to the areas of the body needing more energy, they must pass through the fat cell membrane. The cell membranes have protein channels that help transport hydrophilic (water soluble) materials in and out of cells, but FFAs and glycerol are able to freely transverse via the lipid-rich bilayer. However, under certain conditions, such as fasting, exercise, and strenuous activity, fat-stored toxins will be released as well.

Fig 2.2

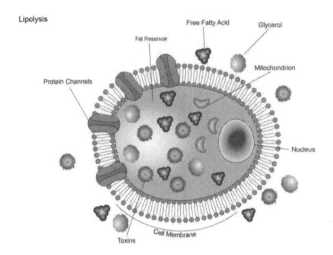

Mobilizing the free fatty acids has been shown to mobilize the lipid-stored pesticides[64, 65] and PCBs[66] in studies.

The release of toxins, such as drug residues, heavy metals, and other xenobiotics from fat cells during extreme lipolysis conditions is the basis to understanding the Hubbard Method. Knowing and proving the principles of the Hubbard Method allowed us to make several breakthroughs for our current protocol.

---

[64] Findlay GM, DeFreitas AS. DDT movement from adipocyte to muscle cell during lipid utilization. Nature. 1971 Jan 1 1971;229(5279):63-65. https://www.nature.com/articles/229063a0.

[65] Mitjavila S, Carrera G, Fernandez Y. Evaluation of the toxic risk of accumulated DDT in the rat: during fat mobilization. Arch Environ Contam Toxicol. 1981 Jul 1981;10(4):471-481. https://www.ncbi.nlm.nih.gov/pubmed/7259309.

[66] de Freitas AS, Norstrom RJ. Turnover and metabolism of polychlorinated biphenyls in relation to their chemical structure and the movement of lipids in the pigeon. Can J Physiol Pharmacol. Dec 1974;52(6):1080-1094. http://www.nrcresearchpress.com/doi/abs/10.1139/y74-142.

How It All Began

The history of our involvement in the Hubbard Method is best told by my father.

Dr. Root: *In September of 1981, I opened up my office in Sacramento, beginning my practice in occupational medicine. Sometime in approximately March of 1982, I was approached by two gentlemen who noted that they had been working as painters approximately one year earlier and were tasked with painting the inside of a 650,000 gallon water tank. They apparently were given no personal protective equipment, including proper masks. They also noted that the inside of the tank became filled with the fumes from their paints and solvents and there was very little ventilation provided to clear the fumes from the large tank. They were exposed to this heavy level of solvent and paint fumes over the period of several days and both became very ill with what I would describe as a toxic encephalopathy. Both men became aggressive, had significant anger control issues resulting in medical problems, problems with short-term memory, and some initial ataxia.*

They had been seen by physicians, but no medications or treatments had been helpful. They did note that there had been some slight improvement, but both their marriages were on the rocks. Their memory problems and feelings of fatigue and emotional lability were still very significant problems for them.

In an attempt to help these men, I went to the medical literature. At that time most of the articles I reviewed indicated that these types of paints and solvents would have a relatively short biologic half-life—in the range of a few hours to perhaps a day or two—at which point, the levels absorbed into the tissue should have decreased by 50%. However, there was little or no information regarding the long term effects from either an extremely heavy exposure, which these men had received, or a lower level exposure over longer periods of time.

At the time I was reviewing the medical literature, I serendipitously received a trifold brochure from a company called "Bodi-Pure," which described a mechanism by which lipid soluble toxicants could be reduced from the body tissues by use of a sauna detoxification program developed by Mr. Hubbard in the late 1960s.

The program used niacin, exercise, heat stress in a sauna, and vitamins and minerals, in an attempt to reduce the body burden of those fat soluble toxic compounds. It piqued my interest, but sounded somewhat simplistic and I tossed the brochure into the trash can! Then it dawned on me that perhaps such a program might be helpful for my two patients, since nothing else seemed to be helping them. After three passes in and out of the waste basket, I finally decided to contact the company and indeed did visit the office, which had been set up in Downtown Sacramento. They provided me with a 4-inch-thick 3-ring binder of medical articles supporting this sauna detoxification program. I was able to borrow the documentation binder over the weekend, read through the entire binder, and was impressed with the scientific basis for this program.

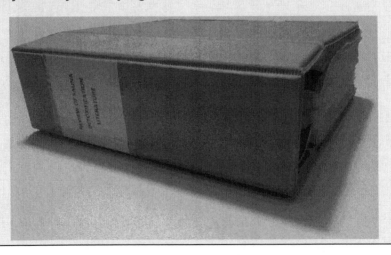

I contacted the two patients and encouraged them to give the program a try. They both went through the program, which required approximately 35 days, 5 hours a day.

They had some significant improvement in their symptoms: fewer headaches, some improvement in their emotional lability/aggressiveness, and no evidence of ataxia.

I cannot say that the program "cured them," but it definitely improved their situation—though not as much as I had hoped. Thinking on this point, I concluded it was likely that if the sauna detoxification program had been started much sooner after the exposure, the improvement would have been more rapid and produced much better results.

After putting these two patients through the sauna detoxification program, I became affiliated with the company and provided pre-treatment physical assessments for their clients and eventually, incorporated the sauna detoxification program into my medical practice under the name HealthMed.

I continued to see a significant number of chemically exposed patients from work exposures; but I also had the opportunity to treat a large number of people who had abused drugs, and could not get off them. Using this sauna detoxification modality proved to be extremely effective. Over the years I estimate that I treated approximately 4,000 patients with this program and found it to be extremely helpful in reducing the body burden of lipid soluble toxic chemicals. More importantly, it improved the symptom complexes which the chemically exposed patients exhibited, thereby improving their quality of life very significantly.

My father is recognized as the leading expert in sauna-based human detoxification, despite the early disregard of his peers, and for repurposing L. Ron Hubbard's Purification Rundown for the treatment of workplace chemical exposure injuries. He is a Christian elder in the Presbyterian Church and has no ties or affiliations with Scientology.

Wikipedia unfortunately has persisted in providing incorrect information in my father's bio, including the error that he is "Known for ... Scientology."[67]

In a 2007 interview with the *Sacramento News and Review*, my father explains, "If you look my name up on the Internet, you would think I was a scientology buff. I am an elder in the Presbyterian Church. I am not a scientologist. ... It's just the fact that, by gosh, Hubbard put this thing together. He deserves recognition for that. ...We have no ties to the Church of Scientology. We're very upfront about how L. Ron Hubbard developed this."[68]

From detox projects around the world, my father and his colleagues have empirically demonstrated an average 42.4% reduction of 16 lipophilic toxins in patients in one study.[69] Another study of First Responders and volunteers of 9/11 measured 65% decreases in PCB toxicity after the Hubbard Method of sauna detoxification.[70]

---

[67] Wikipedia contributors, "David Emerson Root," Wikipedia, The Free Encyclopedia, https://en.wikipedia.org/w/index.php?title=David_Emerson_Root&oldid=854392411 (accessed December 16, 2018).

[68] Gianni, Luke. "Scientology does detox." *Sacramento News & Review*, February 22, 2007. https://www.newsreview.com/sacramento/scientology-does-detox/content?oid=283982.

[69] Prousky, ND, MSc, Jonathan E. "Niacin for Detoxification: A Little-known Therapeutic Use." *JOM* 26, no. 2 (2011), 85-92. http://ionhealth.ca/wp-content/uploads/resources/PDFs/Niacin-for-Detoxification-A-Little-known-Therapeutic-Use-26.2.pdf.

[70] Dahlgren J , et al. "Persistent Organic Pollutants in 9/11 World Trade Center Rescue Workers: Reduction Following Detoxification. - PubMed - NCBI." National Center for Biotechnology Information. https://www.ncbi.nlm.nih.gov/pubmed/17234251.

Subjectively these reductions translated to 78-100% improvement in reported symptoms, on average.

We will explore a few case studies beginning on page 78.

Don't Just Detox, *Get Detoxinated!*™

In 2014, I began to develop this medical detoxification protocol into a health and wellness program, and it was rolled out in December of 2017. We trademarked the word *Detoxination®* to differentiate our preventive/wellness therapy from detoxification. This updated protocol reduces the time commitment from 30 days down to just 14 (or less), and from 4-5 hours per day down to around two.

We now offer both a medically supervised and a wellness version of Detoxination. From a medical history and symptom survey, the determination is made as to which protocol is most appropriate. Medically supervised Detoxination involves physicals, lab tests, medical staff interactions, staff review of daily vitals and log sheets, and approximately 30 days "on program."

Detoxination addresses nutrition, detoxification, and toxin avoidance unlike any other program available. Nutrition and toxin avoidance will be discussed in greater detail later in this book. Sauna detoxification will be the focus of this chapter, once we get a few key concepts out of the way:

- Toxic material that was sequestered away in fat cells tends to remain lodged there for many years unless and until acted upon.
- Lipophilic xenobiotics, or toxins that readily bond with fat, can induce inflammation by a variety of different mechanisms, many of which result in cell injury, degeneration, and/or the death of most or all of the cells in

an organ or tissue due to disease, injury, or failure of the blood supply.

- "Lipolysis" is a naturally occurring process in which fat cells are broken down, usually during fasting and exercise, to release stored energy. This breakdown also mobilizes Free Fatty Acids (FFAs), glycerol and, more importantly, toxins back into the bloodstream.

- Mobilization of xenobiotics is not desirable if routes of elimination are not simultaneously enhanced.

- Chemicals are excreted through many routes including feces, urine, sweat, sebum (an oily secretion of the sebaceous glands), and lung vapor.

Exercise

As fat is stored throughout the body with significant deposits in adipose and brain tissues, exercise is aimed at both promoting deep circulation in the tissues and enhancing the turnover of fats.

It is well known that exercise promotes the circulation of blood to tissues, but it also promotes mobilization of lipids from storage depots. As we have demonstrated, mobilization of the fat stores is accompanied by mobilization of the toxins stored in the fatty tissue.

The goal of exercise, therefore, is to distribute the mobilized toxins, via increased blood circulation, to the routes of elimination in the dermis layers which lead to sweat (more on this to follow).

Low impact aerobic exercises from an exercycle, treadmill, an elliptical machine, or jogging, is done at the beginning of each session. Exercise is gradually increased to 20-30 minutes—depending on individual fitness level—and kept in a Training Heart Rate (THR) range for both blood circulation and fat burn.

In the lower intensity THR "fat-burning zone," the body relies on more stored fat (versus carbs) as its primary fuel source compared to a higher intensity workout. The formula to calculate your THR range is provided on page 134.

After calculating the upper and lower THR range, monitor your heart rate during exercise. A FitBit or similar device is recommended.

Sauna

The purpose of the sauna aspect of the program is threefold: increasing circulation via heat stress, increasing lipolysis (mobilization), and enhancing the elimination of compounds through both sweat and sebum (explained momentarily).

Skin, the largest organ of the body, averages around 20 square feet in area and weighs approximately 6 pounds. Skin is classified as an organ because it sends and receives messages to other parts of the body. It is also your first line of defense against environmental elements including bacteria, chemicals, heavy metals, some gases, and even the sun's rays.

During any program in which toxins are deliberately mobilized from fat stores, it is important that elimination keep pace with this mobilization process. Otherwise, it is possible that mobilization will result in heightened blood concentrations of the circulating compounds, thus causing further complications.

The safest and most effective means of toxicant elimination has long been found via sweat from sauna usage. For more information on the history of sauna and how to build your own, pick up a copy of *The Holistic Handbook of Sauna Therapy* by Nenah Sylver, PhD.

There are two types of sweat produced by glands in the skin. One of the glands is the sudoriferous sweat gland, which produces 99%

water and 1% salt to cool the body. The other is called the sebaceous gland, which produces an oily sebum used to coat the hair follicle and seal moisture in to prevent hair from breaking and skin from cracking. There are approximately 90 of these sebaceous glands per square inch of skin. It is through the sebaceous sweat that many waste products (including bacteria and xenobiotics) are excreted during strenuous activities or high heat levels, as attained during sauna.

Although regular sweat can release minute traces of toxins, sebaceous sweat is the main goal of sauna detoxification. See Figure 2.3 for a cut-away view of a skin section with the sweat gland and sebaceous oil gland illustrated.

Fig. 2.3

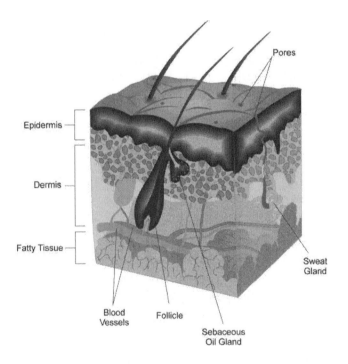

Unless otherwise noted, when we use the term "sweat" from now on, we mean the combination of regular sweat and sebaceous sweat.

Many heavy metals, methadone, amphetamines, methamphetamines and morphine, and other compounds appear in human sweat.[71, 72] Sebum-rich sebaceous sweat has been shown to contain high concentrations of PCBs.[86] Enhancement of this elimination is a key purpose of the sauna.

In addition to an increase in sweat production, increased body temperature from sauna usage results in heightened production of toxin-laced sebum from the sebaceous glands.

With the right kind of sauna and conditions, even greater quantities of toxic material can be excreted via sebaceous sweat. In our centers, we only use and promote Full Spectrum Infrared Saunas manufactured by Clearlight Infrared® makers of Jacuzzi® infrared saunas for maximum yield.

Infrared rays are one of the sun's rays and are the healthiest. They'll penetrate into your skin deeply, and they dissolve harmful substances accumulated in your body. The infrared light rays vitalize your cells and metabolism.

Full spectrum refers to the entire infrared spectrum: near infrared, mid or medium infrared, and far infrared.

---

[71] "Arsenic, Cadmium, Lead, and Mercury in Sweat: A Systematic Review." Hindawi. Last modified February 22, 2012. https://www.hindawi.com/journals/jeph/2012/184745/.
[72] "Excretion of Methamphetamine and Amphetamine in Human Sweat Following Controlled Oral Methamphetamine Administration." PubMed Central (PMC). https://www.ncbi.nlm.nih.gov/pmc/articles/PMC2714868/.

Near infrared is the shortest wavelength and will be absorbed just below the surface of the skin, thus creating conditions that promote cell healing and revitalization.

Mid infrared is a longer wavelength that can penetrate deeper into the body's soft tissue, thus increasing circulation and releasing oxygen to reach injured areas and reduce pain.

Far infrared is the longest wavelength that penetrates the fat cells, thus causing vasodilation. The fat cells vibrate to expel toxins, resulting in the greatest levels of detoxification. Far infrared has the reputation of stimulating the metabolism and aiding in weight loss.

Among the infrared waves, the far infrared rays, which have a longer wavelength, are especially good for the human body. These waves have the potential to penetrate 1.5 to 2 inches or more into the body, allowing for deeper heat to raise the core body temperature.

The following chart summarizes the claimed benefits of full spectrum infrared wavelengths:

Therapeutic Benefits of Infrared Frequencies			
	Near IR	Mid IR	Far IR
Cellular Health	●		
Wound Healing	●		
Skin Rejuvenation	●		
Pain Relief	●	●	
Improved Micro-circulation		●	
Weight Loss		●	●
Detoxification			●
Blood Pressure Reduction			●
Relaxation			●

Traditional "dry heat" or "dry" saunas are less efficient than infrared because they must first heat the surrounding air (convection) before warming the body (conduction).

In a presentation at the Biological Medicine 2012 Conference hosted by the Klinghardt Academy in New York City, Dr. Dietrich Klinghardt reported on a study he conducted to find just how dramatic the difference in detoxification is between conventional and infrared saunas. Dr. Klinghardt, who is considered an authority on the subject of metal toxicity and its connection with chronic infections, illness and pain, said lab results showed that the sweat of people using a conventional sauna was 95-97 percent water while the sweat of those using an infrared thermal system was 80-85 percent water. The remaining 15-20% non-water portion is sebaceous sweat containing cholesterol, fat soluble toxins, toxic heavy metals, sulfuric acid, sodium, ammonia, and uric acid.

In our Centers, individuals spend a total of 75 minutes, on average, over two sauna cycles. The first sauna cycle is typically 45 minutes (or as tolerated), and after a 15 minute cool-down to prevent heat exhaustion, another 30 minutes will be spent in the sauna.

During the cool down, a cold shower to wash off excreted toxins is recommended to prevent reabsorption through the pores. However, toweling can accomplish the task and provides an opportunity to "dry brush" your skin to stimulate the lymphatic system. Just remember to always brush or towel yourself towards your heart!

Oils, Binders, and Supplementation

During the Protocol, minerals, vitamins, and electrolytes are administered. These balance the niacin intake and replenish the nutrients and fluids lost to sweat.

Cold pressed, polyunsaturated oils are also provided. Rich in essential fatty acids, the oils may be a blend of organic hemp, walnut, flaxseed and/or sunflower oil.

These oils tend to prevent enterohepatic recirculation (reprocessing in the liver) of the mobilized toxic material by coating the intestinal lining to block reabsorption and increase the excretion rate of certain lipophilic compounds in the bile.[73] Polyunsaturated oils have been found to replace niacin-mobilized lipids in adipose tissue stores in a lipid exchange mechanism.[73] Additionally, these oils enhance the excretion of extremely persistent chemicals without depositing fat in the liver. They are necessary for cell-membrane function and they provide an excellent balance of omega 3 and omega 6 essential fatty acids to improve health.

Each day of the protocol, we mix up to 4 tablespoons (as tolerated) of the selected oils into a small glass or Dixie cup to drink after exercising. Adding a shot of 100% organic cranberry juice improves the taste.

Lecithin is recommended during the protocol as it is the major dietary source of choline, a semi-essential nutrient that is part of the B-complex vitamin family. Choline is essential in lipid metabolism and cell membrane structure, and it can help transport fat soluble drugs and nutrients across fat insoluble cell membranes.

Binders such as Bentonite clay, zeolite clay, and activated charcoal (AC) also reduce risks from enterohepatic recirculation and overwhelming the liver.

A complete sample daily routine, with timing and recommended amounts of oils, and binders begins on page 121.

Included in the protocol is a complete list of vitamins and minerals needed to replenish those lost through sweating and to correct

---

[73] Rea, William J. "35 Thermal Chamber Depuration and Physical Therapy." In *Chemical Sensitivity: Tools, Diagnosis and Method of Treatment, Volume IV*, 1st ed., 2459. Boca Raton: Taylor & Francis, 1996. ISBN-13: 978-0873719650

deficiencies. This can be especially important for the fat soluble vitamins (A, D, E, K). Vitamin A, for example, undergoes extensive enterohepatic recirculation and must be supplemented at higher than normal doses as increased fecal excretion is likely.[74]

The general topic of vitamin and mineral supplementation is too overarching for this tome. I can tell you, however, that the original research, as well as decades of real-world experience, have produced a working vitamin and mineral replenishment schedule (included in Chapter 3), which increases proportionately with niacin doses as the protocol progresses.

Good vitamins and minerals should be sourced from suppliers that do not use fillers, colors, or preservatives. Watch for GMO ingredients as well.

Two of the most important minerals, calcium and magnesium, are consumed separately from the other supplements in a beverage known as Cal-Mag.

Calcium is a basic building block in the body, and its deficiency from sweating sets up muscle spasms. Both calcium and magnesium are helpful in relieving sore muscles.

Magnesium provides a relaxing, antioxidant and anti-inflammatory effect. It is critical for over 300 metabolic processes, cell growth, and reproduction. Magnesium is involved in hundreds of enzyme processes affecting every aspect of life. It is not only essential for maintaining good health, but also for detoxification and the treatment of numerous diseases.

---

[74] Sodhi, H.S., Wood, P.D.S., Schlierf, G. and Kinse11, L.W., Plasma, Bile and Fecal Sterols in Relation to Diet,Metabolism 16: 4:334-344, 1967. https://www.metabolismjournal.com/article/0026-0495(67)90045-5/pdf.

If you sweat to the point that you develop a magnesium deficiency, you may experience a variety of symptoms. These include feelings of anxiety and irritability, difficulty sleeping, low blood pressure, confusion, muscle weakness, spasms and hyperventilation.

The protocol causes profuse sweating which results in an excessive loss of both calcium and magnesium. Therefore, it is essential to drink at least one glass of the Cal-Mag formula during each session.

The Cal-Mag recipe of calcium gluconate, magnesium carbonate, and apple cider vinegar is also found on page 126. It is extremely important to follow the instructions carefully if you wish to drink a pleasant, more palatable mix!

Hydration and Electrolytes

A person can lose more than 2 liters per hour of fluids to sweat during each session; therefore, it is vital to keep hydrated with filtered water. Distilled water is not recommended for rehydration.[75] Similarly, coconut water is high in potassium, but it is unable to hydrate as effectively as purified water.

Your goal should be to consume as much water as you sweat out. Simply weigh yourself before you begin your session, and then record your weight again at the end. The deviation will reveal if you either drank too little or too much (preferred). Remember the protocol may have a weight loss benefit; however, this is only apparent after you complete your Detoxination Program!

Electrolytes, in the form of sodium chloride (salt), cell salts, and potassium should be available to replenish electrolytes lost to sweat. Symptoms of electrolyte depletion are similar to heat exhaustion,

---

[75] "Early Death Comes From Drinking Distilled Water." Mercola.com. https://www.mercola.com/article/water/distilled_water.htm.

including clammy skin, weakness or extreme tiredness, headaches, nausea, cramps, vomiting, and fainting. It is recommended to take electrolytes, as directed, after each sauna session.

Niacin (aka Nicotinic Acid or Vitamin B3)

It is important to understand that **niacin is the key to successful sauna detoxification.** Niacin can shift the fat/blood equilibrium of toxic concentrations by stimulating lipolysis release of fatty acids from the fat cells into the bloodstream.

In order to achieve the desired rate and quantity of xenobiotics released from fats, the protocol exploits a little known property of nicotinic acid to trigger a state called "rebound lipolysis." Once ingested, niacin has a short-term effect of *reducing* the lipolysis mobilization of free fatty acids for approximately 2.5 hours. When the short-term niacin effect subsides, a transitory — yet substantial — increase in mobilized FFAs, glycerol, and toxins follows.

Picture dangling a rubber band from your pinched fingers to represent normal lipolysis and then stretched vertically to simulate the lipolysis decrease from niacin. When the bottom of the loop is released (representing the waning niacin effect) the rubber band shoots up into the air as it *rebounds* with kinetic energy.

As reported in a 1969 study on this niacin effect in both sheep and humans,

> The elevation of total FFA turnover during the rebound phase indicates that the elevation of plasma FFA level is due to increased mobilization of fatty acids, presumably from adipose tissue triglycerides, and is not the result of decreased utilization. Support for the view that the rising plasma FFA level in the rebound phase was due to increased lipolysis is

provided by the increasing plasma glycerol level, since glycerol that results from complete hydrolysis of triglycerides is not available for reesterification within adipose tissue.[76]

Once the state of rebound lipolysis begins, after 2.5 to 3 hours (depending on dose, food intake, and other factors), the fat cells increase their lipolysis output of FFAs, glycerol, <u>and toxins</u> by a striking 200%[77]!

This is the science *and magic* behind Detoxination!

[76] Nye, E. R., and Hilaire Buchanan. "Short-term effect of nicotinic acid on plasma level and turnover of free fatty acids in sheep and man." *Journal of Lipid Research* 10, no. 2 (1969), 193-6. http://www.jlr.org/content/10/2/193.long.

[77] Wang W, et al. "Effects of Nicotinic Acid on Fatty Acid Kinetics, Fuel Selection, and Pathways of Glucose Production in Women. - PubMed - NCBI." National Center for Biotechnology Information. https://www.ncbi.nlm.nih.gov/pubmed/10893322.

Rebound lipolysis can average four hours as illustrated in Figure 2.4.

Fig 2.4

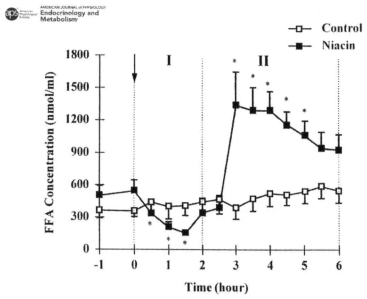

Plasma free fatty acid (FFA) concentrations in response to chronic and acute nicotinic acid (NA) or control.
* $P < 0.05$ vs. control. Arrow denotes time of NA administration.

Published in: Wei Wang; Alice Basinger; Richard A. Neese; Mark Christiansen; Marc K. Hellerstein; *American Journal of Physiology-Endocrinology and Metabolism* **2000**, 279, E50-E59.
DOI: 10.1152/ajpendo.2000.279.1.E50

It is during this period of rebound lipolysis that the protocol is most effective. A standard session only requires two hours, preferably at the peak of the rebound (or three hours after ingesting niacin).

Other studies have confirmed the rebound effect and also shed light on a Target Niacin Dose (TND) between 500mg[76] (at the low end) and a maximum of 10mg/kg to achieve the desired response.[78]

---

[78] Pereira, Joseph N. "The plasma free fatty acid rebound induced by nicotinic acid." *Journal of Lipid Research* 8, no. 3 (May 1967), 239-44.
http://www.jlr.org/content/8/3/239.full.pdf.

Figure 2.5 depicts the increased volume of FFAs, glycerol, and toxins.

Fig. 2.5

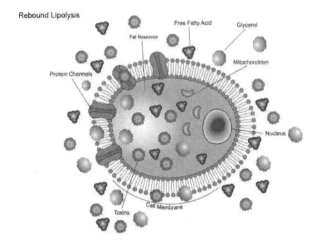

This 200% increased release of FFAs is measurable, as noted in Fig. 2.5. And a corresponding increase in blood serum levels of toxins is also well documented in the literature.[70] Once in the blood, these mobilized toxins must be quickly ushered to the dermis by exercise to be excreted in sauna-induced sweat or captured in the GI tract by binders.

The research confirming the rebound lipolysis effect was the key to shortening and amending the original Hubbard protocol and creating refinements that became the Detoxination Protocol. We also discovered that using a different type of sauna—full spectrum infrared—improved the outcome. The initial protocol had begun with the niacin dose, after which patients exercised for 20-30 minutes. This was followed by multiple sauna cycles averaging only 15-25 minutes each, due to the oppressive heat, for the remaining four hours.

At our Detoxination Wellness Centers we understand how to exploit rebound lipolysis. Our clients ingest their niacin dose 2 hours prior to their arrival at the Centers. By the time they have recorded their vitals and changed into suitable attire, they have reached the desired state of rebound lipolysis.

An equally important function of niacin, unrelated to potential mobilization of lipophilic toxins, is the synthesis of nicotinamide adenine dinucleotide phosphate (NADPH) required to regenerate reduced glutathione[79]. Glutathione is a water soluble antioxidant that plays an important role in Phase II detoxification processes.

No other form of niacin, like niacinimide, inositol, or hexaniacinate, has the same biological properties that will trigger rebound lipolysis. Only Immediate Release (IR) niacin is used in this program since Sustained Released (SR) niacin can cause liver toxicity. This is almost never seen with IR, or pure crystalline niacin.

The pure crystalline form of niacin is preferred over the convenient pills or capsules. The crystalline form dissolves and reacts faster, and switching from one form to another can cause nausea.

The administration of niacin causes a rather uncomfortable flushing or reddening of the skin of the arms, legs and body with an itchy or prickly sensation, which occurs approximately 10 to 45 minutes after ingestion. Though uncomfortable, this vasodilation effect helps to significantly increase blood circulation to the dermis layers, thereby enhancing the removal of xenobiotics during sauna.

The target niacin dose (TND), which is calculated at 10mg per kilogram of body weight, [63] is titrated up in the first 5-7 days, or as

---

[79] Klaidman LK, Mukherjee SK, Adams JDJ. Oxidative changes in brain pyridine nucleotides and neuroprotection using nicotinamide. Biochim Biophys Acta. 2001 Feb 16 2001;1525(1-2):136-148. https://www.ncbi.nlm.nih.gov/pubmed/11342263.

tolerated. Warning: Before taking any supplement, especially in doses above Recommended Daily Allowances, you should consult with your medical professional.

The initial niacin dose should be 50-100 mg. Most people can tolerate 100mg increments. For many, this may bring you up to your TND in 10-11 days. If you find that you can tolerate 200-300 mg/day increases during that 10 days, by all means, do so!

The TND has been demonstrated[77] to produce the ideal rebound lipolysis as seen in Fig 1. Taking excessively large niacin doses potentially delays the start of the rebound effect (sometimes by several hours), decreases the volume of released substances, or reduces the duration of the rebound effect.

After reaching your TND, continue to incrementally increase your daily dose. The body builds up a tolerance to niacin[80] during the protocol; therefore, it is necessary to continually provide more niacin to achieve the desired rebound. 200-300 mg/day increases are more tolerable after reaching 1,000 mg (1 g), but always stay at or below 5 g. Most will average 3,000-3,500 mg on the program.

Completion

When to stop the protocol is a question without a definitive answer. It will depend on the individual variables found in Chapter 1. One thing is for certain, most everyone has a sense for the point in which they have achieved an "End Phenomenon." This is completely subjective, but it has been described as the point where an individual sees improvement in both their physical and mental well-being.

---

[80] Stern, Ralph H., J. D. Spence, David J. Freeman, and Anwar Parbtani. "Tolerance to nicotinic acid flushing." *Clinical Pharmacology and Therapeutics* 50, no. 1 (1991), 66-70. https://www.ncbi.nlm.nih.gov/pubmed/1855354.

People report being more mentally alert and aware, looking and feeling remarkably better, and sleeping more soundly. It is our experience that most will not get there until around day 14, and it can even take 30 days or more.

During the protocol, several interesting manifestations may occur that you should not be alarmed by. Niacin has a histamine-like effect on the skin caused by vasodilation. Many people report seeing old sunburns appearing on their body in the shape or design of past swimwear. Others have noted swelling where old injuries once were, after which the swelling disappears forever within a brief period. These manifestations should be documented if you have volunteered to participate in our *Get Detoxinated!*™ program explained later in this book.

Even more common are sensations, smells, and tastes from past experiences with certain chemicals, fragrances, drugs, foods, smoke, and other substances. Additionally, sweat can produce colorful stains from various chemicals (this will be addressed on page 132).

Upon cessation of the detox protocol, continue taking niacin in decrementing doses to taper down from such high levels. It is not unreasonable to reduce your daily intake 300-500mg/day, and you do not need to completely stop niacin as it has many health benefits. The RDA is 16mg/day for males, and 14mg/day for women who aren't pregnant.

Continue with the vitamins and minerals accordingly, as well. Your body is healing, so keep feeding it the necessary materials to properly rebuild.

The Hubbard Method was specifically developed to reduce the levels of drug residues. However, it has proven to be applicable to the reduction of other fat stored compounds as well. Over the last decade this program has gained widespread support due to its effectiveness and the fact that it is well supported by the medical literature. When utilizing the methodology described herein, analysis of blood concentrations of xenobiotics during treatment has shown that excretion keeps pace with the levels of xenobiotics mobilized from fat stores[81].

Dr. Root: *The sauna detoxification program was designed to lower the body burden of fat soluble chemicals, but as it turns out, it also reduces levels of water-soluble xenobiotics. Because of this, the sauna detoxification program is a very formidable instrument for reducing the body burden of many compounds.*

Based on my observations, 85 percent of the toxins are excreted through the sweat and about 15 percent are excreted through the gastrointestinal tract.

As far as I can determine from an extensive review of the literature over the past 36 years, there is no known program which even comes close to doing what this program can do for people so exposed.

Can Toxins Really Be Eliminated In Sweat?

We have seen very misleading articles and videos that dispute the ability of sauna detoxification to produce significant quantities of toxin-laden sweat. First, these hit pieces never address sebum-rich sebaceous sweat, only liquid sweat. Second, they don't mention mobilizing toxins via niacin-induced rebound lipolysis.

Then there is the word "toxins," which they use to obfuscate the real problem of lipophilic xenobiotics such as heavy metals, synthetic

---

[81] Schnare DW and Robinson PC. "Reduction of the Human Body Burdens of Hexachlorobenzene and Polychlorinated Biphenyls. - PubMed - NCBI." National Center for Biotechnology Information. https://www.ncbi.nlm.nih.gov/pubmed/3110064.

chemicals, and persistent organic pollutants. We refer to these as "toxins" for simplicity sake as well, but I want to emphasize that not all toxins are of the water soluble kind that your natural detox organs can easily handle. The most dangerous toxins are fat soluble, and the sources of misinformation never make this distinction.

Attempts to knock sauna detox are further misleading because they only address the companies that provide a 1-2 hour sauna session—not the 2-week niacin-based, scientifically proven protocol we have been using to save lives for over 35 years!

Moreover, we have never seen these debunkers produce scientific, peer-reviewed research papers to support their claims. But we do in this book![82]

In their book *Beyond Antibiotics*, Drs. Michael A. Schmidt et al. state the following: "Saunas are being used by some doctors to stimulate the release of toxins from the bodies of their patients. They have found that a lower temperature (105-110 Fahrenheit) sauna taken for a longer duration is most beneficial. These low temperatures stimulate a fat [sebaceous] sweat, which eliminates toxins stored in fat, as opposed to the high temperature sauna, which encourages a water sweat."[83]

Arsenic, cadmium, lead, and mercury have been shown in studies[84] to be excreted through the skin as well as—or better—than in urine. Another study[85] found BPA in 80% of the subjects' sweat while

---

[82] See the Response Letter to the Medical Board of California on page 174

[83] Schmidt, Michael A., Lendon H. Smith, and Keith W. Sehnert. *Beyond Antibiotics: 50 (or so) Ways to Boost Immunity and Avoid Antibiotics*. Berkeley, Calif: North Atlantic Books, 1994.

[84] "Arsenic, Cadmium, Lead, and Mercury in Sweat: A Systematic Review." Hindawi. https://www.hindawi.com/journals/jeph/2012/184745/.

[85] "Human Excretion of Bisphenol A: Blood, Urine, and Sweat (BUS) Study." PubMed Central (PMC). https://www.ncbi.nlm.nih.gov/pmc/articles/PMC3255175/.

finding no detectable levels in their blood or urine. Sweat is the ideal way to remove certain carcinogenic PCBs[86], PBDEs (found in flame retardants)[87], phthalates[88], and volatile organic hydrocarbons.

Key findings in a study[56] on human elimination of phthalate compounds, DEHP (di (2-ethylhexl) phthalate) and MEHP (mono(2-ethylhexyl) phthalate), include:

- DEHP and/or its metabolite MEHP were found in all participants, suggesting that exposure to potentially toxic phthalate compounds is very common.
- Some parent phthalate compounds and some metabolites were apparently readily excreted in sweat; others were not.
- In several individuals, DEHP was found in sweat but not in serum, suggesting the possibility of some degree of phthalate retention and bioaccumulation.
- Some toxic phthalate metabolites such as MEHP were eliminated comparatively well in sweat.

In short, sweating can be one of the cheapest, safest and most effective ways to detoxify.

Case Studies

Between 1982 and 2007, my father was working with many detoxification projects around the world involving Dr. George Yu and

[86] Genuis SJ, Beesoon S, Birkholz D. Biomonitoring and Elimination of Perfluorinated Compounds and Polychlorinated Biphenyls through Perspiration: Blood, Urine, and Sweat Study. ISRN Toxicol. 2013;2013:483832. Published 2013 Sep 3. https://www.ncbi.nlm.nih.gov/pmc/articles/PMC3776372/.

[87] Genuis SK, Birkholz D, Genuis SJ. Human Excretion of Polybrominated Diphenyl Ether Flame Retardants: Blood, Urine, and Sweat Study. Biomed Res Int. 2017;2017:3676089. https://www.ncbi.nlm.nih.gov/pmc/articles/PMC5360950/.

[88] Genuis SJ, Beesoon S, Lobo RA, Birkholz D. Human elimination of phthalate compounds: blood, urine, and sweat (BUS) study. ScientificWorldJournal. 2012;2012:615068. https://www.ncbi.nlm.nih.gov/pmc/articles/PMC3504417/.

a coalition of physicians, researchers, environmentalists, scientists, and educators for the Foundation for Advancements in Science and Education (FASE), a Los Angeles company that provided support of the detox programs.

Two peer-reviewed studies, involving my father's participation, were published: the New York Rescue Workers Detoxification Project,[70] which ran from 2002-2007, and the Utah Meth Cops Project, which began in October 2007 and concluded in July 2010.[89]

A third study on veterans suffering a condition known as Gulf War Syndrome concluded in 2015 with promising subjective results; however, final release date of the empirical data is unknown. Its purpose was to evaluate the ability of rehabilitative therapy to decrease the symptoms and improve the quality of life of Gulf War Veterans who suffer from Gulf War Illness. The study results were submitted July 31, 2018, but remain unpublished at the time of this writing.

Although these results may someday become available, the fact that the government even awarded the Gulf War Syndrome Study in September 2010, is truly remarkable.

Gulf War illness is found in about one fourth of veterans of the 1990-1991 Gulf War and is characterized by persistent memory and concentration problems, headaches, fatigue, and muscle and joint pain. It is not known what causes the illness, but exposure to chemicals is suspected.

---

[89] Ross GH, Sternquist MC. Methamphetamine exposure and chronic illness in police officers: significant improvement with sauna-based detoxification therapy. *Toxicol Ind Health*. 2012;28(8):758-68.
https://www.ncbi.nlm.nih.gov/pmc/articles/PMC3573677/.

The Gulf War Syndrome Study—titled *Gulf War Illness –Evaluation of an innovative detoxification program*—was the product of more than a decade-long series of presentations to Congress, the Department of Defense, and the CDC. An important quote from the testimony given by my father to the Presidential Special Oversight Board for Department of Defense Investigations of Gulf War Chemical & Biological Incidents in 1998 was published in Dr. Nenah Sylver's book, *The Holistic Handbook of Sauna Therapy*,

> Since 1982, I have been using a detoxification program to treat patients who have been exposed to fat soluble chemicals, either at work or from environmental sources. This program, developed by L. Ron Hubbard in 1978, has over the last 15 years been evaluated and used by a growing number of professionals throughout the world who have examined its use in relieving the after effects of chemical exposure and found it to be very effective. To my knowledge, there is no other peer-reviewed method for reducing the body burden of fat soluble toxic chemicals. Papers documenting the efficacy of the Hubbard program have been published by such organizations as the World Health Organization, the Royal Swedish Academy of Science, the Society for Occupational and Environmental Health and others....The Hubbard detoxification program has long been upheld as compensable under state and national workman's compensation laws.

His full testimony, along with the transcript of the entire proceedings, is available online.[90]

---

[90] Department Of Defense. *The Presidential Special Oversight Board For Department of Defense Investigations of Gulf War Chemical & Biological Incidents*. Senate Hart Building, Washington, DC, 1998.
https://gulflink.health.mil/oversight/frid.htm#p116.

> **Dr. Root:** *The Gulf War Veterans from the first Gulf War were exposed to multiple chemicals, including smoke from oil fires, and pyridostigmine bromide tablets, used to protect them against nerve-agent attacks. Also much of the clothing used during that portion of the war was impregnated with DEET, and permethrin. Many, if not most of the veterans, were also given anthrax vaccine. Symptoms consisted of headaches, fatigue, memory problems, irritability, lack of energy, sleep problems, and joint muscle and tendon pains— particularly in the shoulders, feet, hands and knees. I treated several of these patients with excellent results: Most felt that the above symptom-complex was at least 90% to 95% improved using the sauna detoxification program.*
>
> *Dr. David Carter, occupational medicine specialist and researcher from New York University in Albany, New York, has recently completed a study of 50 Gulf War veterans and his study results should be available in the near future.*[91]

Utah Meth Cops project

When newly elected Utah Attorney General Mark Shurtleff entered his first term in 2000, little did he know that his state was notorious as a leader in the country for the most meth labs per capita. Cops assigned to bust these labs were more concerned about weapons and conducting successful raids than with the dangers from the toxic chemicals used to make methamphetamine. Therefore, protective gear wasn't required, and it may have interfered with their duties. The exposures to these occupational hazards led to the deaths, terminal illnesses, or debilitating symptoms of 81 police officers during the 1980s.

---

[91] Gulf War Illness: Evaluation of an Innovative Detoxification Program. http://cdmrp.army.mil/search.aspx?LOG_NO=GW093066.

Mark Shurtleff learned of the Hubbard Protocol from the New York Rescue Workers Detoxification Project and reached out to FASE. He was able to raise funds to provide sauna detoxification to 68 officers, who suffered from severe acid reflux, heartburn, headaches, spasms, joint pain, insomnia, extreme fatigue, cognitive dysfunction, and various other ailments. A research study recorded this project.

In 2012, a peer-reviewed report of the findings from the Utah Meth Cops Project was published on PubMed.Gov of the US National Library of Medicine for the National Institute of Health (NIH). The report concludes, "This investigation strongly suggests that utilizing sauna and nutritional therapy may alleviate chronic symptoms appearing after chemical exposures associated with methamphetamine-related law enforcement activities. This report also has relevance to addressing the apparent ill effects of other complex chemical exposures. In view of the positive clinical outcomes in this group, broader investigation of this sauna-based treatment regimen appears warranted."[89]

Agent Orange

The U.S. military dumped some 20 million gallons of Agent Orange (2,4,D; 2,4,5,T and dioxins) and other herbicides on about a quarter of former South Vietnam between 1962 and 1971, decimating about 5 million acres of forest to remove the foliage that concealed enemy fighters. Dioxins in Agent Orange have since been linked to birth defects, cancers and other ailments. Thousands of Viet Nam war veterans became ill due to their exposure to this defoliant.

> **Dr. Root:** *The deadly chemical dioxin found in the military defoliant Agent Orange and used during the Vietnam War, poisoned thousands that were exposed to it, including the American servicemen.*

> *Agent orange is composed of a mixture of 2,4,D and 2,4,5-T, both very potent herbicides which contain small amounts of very toxic dioxins and dibenzofurans. Many thousands of troops as well as the Vietnamese citizens were exposed to these chemicals over the latter part of the Vietnam War with multiple symptoms but without effective treatment. I have treated a small number of these patients in my office with excellent results. Years later a cardiologist conducted tests on a person who had been exposed to this chemical but subsequently completed the Hubbard program.*
>
> *He found that the patient's level of dioxin had reduced by 29 percent immediately after the program and an astounding 97 percent eight months later. And all previous symptoms attributed to this poisoning had disappeared.*
>
> *In 2012 a sauna detoxification treatment program was set up in Vietnam which is very successfully treating Vietnamese patients.[92]*

PCB Exposures In Shreveport

In 1987, a fire broke out in a transformer room at the Louisiana State University School of Medicine in Shreveport. Dozens of firefighters became alarmed that they had been exposed to high levels of polychlorinated biphenyls (PCBs). After repeated medical complaints, FASE was contacted for assistance. As the Senior Medical Coordinator, my father evaluated 33 fire fighters for detoxification.

---

[92] *Agent Orange: Vietnam Tests Scientology -Linked Detox Program*. AmEmbassy Hanoi: Unclassified U.S. Department of State Case No. F-2015-05717 Doc No. C05949205, 2017.
https://foia.state.gov/searchapp/DOCUMENTS/FOIA_May2017/F-2015-05717/DOC_0C05949205/C05949205.pdf.

> **Dr. Root:** *In 1987, I was asked to assist the Shreveport City physician in evaluating approximately 33 fire fighters who had been exposed to PCB-containing smoke at a University of Shreveport Electrical Substation. The fire fighters had many of the same symptoms as noted in the Gulf War Syndrome patients, including fatigue, tiredness, some short-term memory problems, dizziness, and some skin irritation problems. Of the 30+ individuals evaluated with physical examinations and fat biopsies for PCB levels, approximately 14 were eventually treated at another facility and had mixed results with treatment.*[93]

PCB Exposures In Semič, Slovenia

Semič, a small town in old Yugoslavia, boasts as its main employer an electrical capacitor manufacturing plant. The capacitors produced at this factory, which employs 1,300 of the roughly 5,000 residents, use PCBs and other lipophilic chemicals in the production line. Personal protective equipment was seldom replaced, and the high production demands precluded the regular use of face masks.

Little thought was given to the toxic hazards these chemicals posed to the workers and their families, so waste was routinely dumped in the surrounding area or burned to produce heat for the factory. Rejected products and surplus PCB barrels were stored in nearby barns, and some farmers even used the oily substance to cover the floors of barns and hoghouses.

Workers began to report diffuse headaches, loss of mental acuity, concentration disabilities, nervousness, sleep disturbances, eye problems (conjunctivitis and light sensitivity), chloracne eruptions and skin rashes, chronic respiratory ailments, gastrointestinal

---

[93] Kilburn KH, Warsaw RH, Shields MG, Neurobehavioral dysfunction in firemen exposed to polychlorinated biphenyls (PCBs): possible improvement after detoxification. Arch Environ Health. 1989; 44:345-50. https://www.ncbi.nlm.nih.gov/pubmed/2514627.

disturbances, paresthesia, joint pains, and edematous swelling of the limbs.

Dr. Root: *Later in 1987, I was also asked to put together a team to go to a small village, approximately 30 miles outside of Ljubljana Yugoslavia (now Slovenia) to evaluate the workers at a capacitor manufacturing plant who had become ill.*

Previously, a 35-year-old woman, whose job consisted of handling the capacitors checking for any PCB oil leaks, had been seen by her physician because of extreme sleepiness (she was sleeping up to 20 hours a day!), extreme fatigue, and though she was not pregnant or lactating, she had been oozing approximately 50 cc of a blue-green fluid from her breasts for several months. Her physician had heard of the detox program and referred her to a clinic, which was then open in the Los Angeles area using the same sauna Detox Program.

She was treated with excellent results: her initial tests showed serum PCB levels of 512 mcg/L but the subcutaneous fat concentration of PCBs was a 102 mg/kg, almost 200 times more than in the serum! Her breast discharge was also evaluated and found to contain 712 mcg/L of PCBs. These levels were the highest of I have ever seen in a living human!

Approximately five days after starting the sauna detoxification, the breast discharge rapidly reduced down to zero. At the end of the treatment, which required approximately 30 days, her serum level had dropped to 338 mcg/L (34% reduction) and the level in her subcutaneous fat had dropped to approximately 39 mg/kg (a 60% reduction).

As a result of her excellent response to the sauna detoxification, the local Government in Slovenia requested that other effected workers in the same capacitor plant be evaluated and possibly treated. We evaluated approximately 24 of the exposed workers and selected 11 for a treatment study.

Thirteen of the 24 served as a control group. This study is unique in that it represents the first controlled study of this detoxification treatment on a group of people who had accumulated high amounts of PCBs.[94]

A treatment facility was located and 11 of these highly exposed men were treated. Though there was some degree of variability, the treatment resulted in a marked improvement in symptoms of the patients while the clinical picture of the control group remained unchanged. Unfortunately, due to political problems, a larger treatment program was never instituted.[11, 12]

Subjective study results are graphed in Figure 2.6.

---

[94] "Occupational, Environmental, And Public Health In Semič: A Case Study Of Polychlorinated Biphenyl (PCB) Pollution." Paper presented at Proceedings/Environmental Impact Analysis Research Council/ASCE, New Orleans, LA, October 11, 1989.
http://citeseerx.ist.psu.edu/viewdoc/download?doi=10.1.1.488.2610&rep=rep1&type=pdf.

Fig. 2.6 - Changes in Self-Rated Severity of Symptoms During Pilot Study

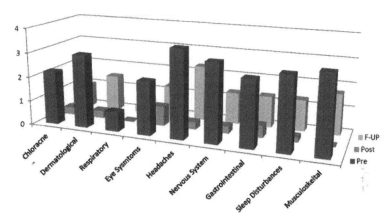

Treated Group (n=11)

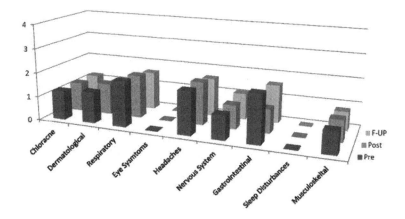

Control Group (n=12)

Patient stated severity of symptoms on a scale of 0 to 5 (0 = none, 1 = slight, 2 = mild, 3 = moderate, 4=severe, and 5 = very severe). Pre, post, and F-up Mean values for each assessment period are plotted. The treated individuals returned to their toxic environment and were re-exposed. Follow-up testing months later showed moderate increases in symptomatology.

2001 New York City Twin Towers Disaster

Dr. Root: *The last large group exposure I would like to discuss in detail is the 09/11/2001 New York City twin towers disaster.*

In October 2001, less than one month after the towers collapsed, my office began receiving phone calls from some of the fire fighters in New York City, who knew of our detoxification program. They were concerned that they were developing serious symptoms from the exposures and were requesting our help.

We put together a team and flew to New York City in January 2002 and conferred with medical personnel from the New York City Fire Department and Police Department, and also with many of the Unions, particularly the EMT Paramedic Union. It soon became clear that no money would be made available for this treatment program, but we were told that if funding could be found, they would welcome our help.

Donated money was sought and found, and a sauna detoxification clinic was opened in lower Manhattan two blocks from Ground Zero in September 2002, just a year after the disaster. Since that time the New York detox unit has treated over 1,000 individuals, primarily first responders, but also some other community members who were extremely sick from the exposure to the dust and fumes.

The response to the sauna detoxification program was nothing short of incredible! Most individuals who were heavily exposed to the dust from the towers and had primarily pulmonary symptoms to begin with, were able to bring up from their tracheo-bronchial tree, large amounts of blackish mucous. Some 30% of those treated had significant amounts of colored material coming out of their skin with their sweat: purple, yellow, black, brown, and grey!

> *This was a somewhat unusual finding since most of the patients whom I had treated previously did not have such heavy particulate exposure. However, in the New York group, most of the first responders had inhaled heavy amounts of particulates and these were not being moved out of the trachea or upper airways by the usual treatment methods. The improvement in these patients was significant. Many of them who had been taken off work and expected to be permanently removed from duty, were allowed to return to duty or at least had significant improvement in their quality of life.*

Following is a summation of the medical folders from 475 men and women who enrolled in the program between 2002 and 2005.

At enrollment, only 14% stated their current health was very good and none stated they were in excellent health. Additionally, 86% of these participants reported their health was poor or fair when they enrolled in the program. At completion 80% stated their health was very good or excellent and six months later 59% of clients still maintained this level of good health.[95]

If the participants had continued access to a sauna for home use, it is likely that the excellent level of health noted at the end of treatment would have been maintained.

Summary of Results

Review of initial test results and medical history questionnaires reveals the following:

---

[95] Cecchini, MS, Marie A., David E. Root, MD, MPH, Jeremie R. Rachunow, MD, and Phyllis M. Gelb, MD. "Chemical Exposures at the World Trade Center: Use of the Hubbard Sauna Detoxification Regimen to Improve the Health Status of New York City Rescue Workers Exposed to Toxicants." *Townsend Letter*, December 2006. http://www.townsendletter.com/Dec2006/chemexp1206.htm.

- All clients reported improvement in subjective symptoms.
- All clients reported improved perception of health.
- Health History and Symptom Survey (selected questions) found considerable reduction in days of work missed on the start of the detoxification program, leading to reduced concerns about forced retirement.
- Due to symptom improvement, 84% of those clients requiring medications to manage symptoms related to WTC exposure were able to discontinue their use.
- Over half the clients required multiple pulmonary medications on entry to achieve near-normal pulmonary functions (measured as FVC & FEV1). On completion of detoxification, 72% of these individuals were free of pulmonary medication yet had improved pulmonary function tests (data not shown).
- There was a statistically significant improvement in thyroid function tests.
- There was a statistically significant improvement in Choice Reaction Time (CRT) and Intelligence Quotient (IQ), suggestive of improvement in cognitive function.
- There was statistically significant improvement in Postural Sway Test, which indicated improvement in vestibular function.

This regimen has greatly reduced the number of work days that rescue workers missed due to illness. It has also resolved anxieties that careers will be ended prematurely due to disability retirement. Anecdotal reports from spouses, family members, and employers describe dramatic changes in the quality of family life as a result of such improvements.

Their subjective results are summarized in Table 2.1:

Table 2.1	Improved At Discharge	Resolved At Discharge
MENTAL HEALTH		
Poor concentration and attention span	12%	84%
Fatigue	14%	82%
Irritability	13%	81%
Impaired memory and mental acuity	20%	78%
Anxiety	12%	88%
Depression	14%	86%
Loss of sleep	16%	80%
Headaches	22%	77%
LUNGS AND AIRWAY		
Sinusitis	9%	91%
Cough	12%	88%
Breathing difficulties	31%	63%
SKIN		
Rash or dryness	24%	70%
MUSCULOSKELETAL		
Joint pain	16%	72%
Muscle pain	19%	79%
Muscle weakness	12%	87%
OTHER		
Increased use of alcohol after 9-11	14%	84%
Eye irritation	12%	78%

The resolution of symptoms at discharge showed *amazing* improvements over pre-treatment surveys!

Five of the patients from the New York Rescue Workers Detoxification Program shared their stories. We have withheld their names for privacy.

Case #1
Paramedic, EMT Trainer, 18-year veteran:

Pre-program – Respiratory problems, lack of energy, loss of concentration, loss of short-term memory, irritability, loss of patience and mood swings. Missed 5-6 weeks of work, faced premature retirement. Two steroids and an inhaler, no improvement.

Day three – No longer needed steroids or inhaler—first time in 10 months.

Day five – *"Pronounced change in my mental ability. Short-term memory improved, attitude and mood much better."*

Week three – *"I was feeling like I did back in my college days; full of energy and mentally sharp. I feel I have benefited tremendously from this program. I feel great physically and sharp mentally. Most importantly, my mood has been uplifted."*

Case #2
Nurse, NYU Downtown, Hospital (33 years):

Pre-program – Chronic lung disease. Heart palpitations. Hyperventilation. Panic attacks. Memory problems (feared early onset of Alzheimer's).

After treatment – Memory returned. Breathing problems resolved. No anxiety. All other issues resolved.

"Before this program, I couldn't walk up the stairs without getting out of breath. Today, I could beat you running down the street."

Case #3
Firefighter, Instructor, Trained 4,200 firefighters:
Pre-program – Unable to sleep more than 2 hours. Nightly nightmares of the event. Breathing difficulties (asthma). No previous illness.

After treatment – *"After a week or two I felt like I was shot out of a cannon, I felt vibrant again. Suddenly I'm sleeping like a baby again, no more nightmares. Mentally and physically almost 100 percent again."*

Case #4
Army Helicopter Pilot:
Became ill Sept 16, 2001.
Remained ill until treatment in Feb 2004.

Pre-program – Chronic nausea, vomiting, diarrhea. Breathing difficulties. Severe stomach and chest pain. Memory problems. Disturbed sleep. Loss of flight privileges. Taking 10 medications. Remaining treatment option: full body steroids.

After treatment – Medication free. Breathing problems resolved. Other symptoms resolved (confirmed by post-treatment evaluation at Walter Reed Medical Center). Regained flight privileges, saving the Army $3,000,000 invested in his training.

"Until just a few weeks ago, I was facing a lifetime of suffering. That is behind me now."

Case #5
Downtown Business Owner:
Pre-program – Chronic lung disease. Chest pains. Rashes. Panic attacks. Joint pain. Taking 14 medications. Unable to work. Remaining treatment option: surgical insertion of iron rod to keep lung inflated.

<u>After treatment</u> – Medication free. Breathing problems resolved. All other issues resolved.

"For the first time in almost 2 years I am taking care of my family and not the other way around. I breathe like a normal human being again. I sleep much better! I am no longer angry or moody. My energy went from less than zero to more than enough!"

For information on other case studies please visit our website at:

https://www.GetDetoxinated.com/case-studies/.

> **Dr. Root:** *An interesting point I'd like to make is that after Detoxination, the body's normal detoxification pathways are greatly improved. The reduction in body burden of most of the lipid soluble toxins continues for months even without further sauna treatment.*[96]

---

[96] Ben, Max. "Is Detoxification A Solution To Occupational Hazards?" *National Safety News,* May 1984.

Toxic Mold and Lyme Disease

Toxic mold poisoning, or mycotoxicosis, can produce upper respiratory symptoms similar to the cold or flu. Mycotoxins are released from mold, which is a type of fungi, for growth and survival. These mycotoxins are a subset of lipophilic biotoxins that are produced by fungal organisms, and are therefore found in fat cells.

Chronic exposures to mycotoxins from mold can cause hair loss, confusion, memory loss, stomach pains, and more. For those with allergies or asthma, more severe symptoms can include headaches, exhaustion, fever, and difficulty breathing. Over time, left untreated, the mycotoxin exposure even be fatal.

These same symptoms parallel Lyme disease. Dr. Neil Nathan has found mold toxicity to be a big piece of the puzzle in a very significant portion of patients with chronic Lyme disease. Dr. Lisa Nagy, who had suffered with mold toxicity herself, has suggested that many Lyme patients have a damaged immune system resulting from mold or pesticide exposures, and that a focus on Lyme and co-infections may not always be the right focus for treatment.[97]

We have had success in treating mold poisoning with this protocol, and we have read many testimonials from others who have received tremendous relief from Lyme disease using this protocol, as well. If you have been diagnosed with Lyme disease or are suffering with mycotoxicosis from mold, we believe this protocol will work synergistically with your current therapy.

---

[97] Forsgren, Scott, Neil Nathan, MD, and Wayne Anderson, ND. "Mold, Mycotoxins, Lyme (July 2014) Townsend Letter for Doctors & Patients." Last modified July 2014. http://www.townsendletter.com/July2014/mold0714_3.html.

WIIFM – What's In It For Me?

The benefits from Detoxination are numerous. I've touched upon some that were reported by our clients and patients, such as:

- Feeling Better/Renewed
- Reduced Aches and Pains
- Improved Overall Health
- Peace of Mind
- Greater Energy
- Better Skin and Body Scent
- Raised Cognition and I.Q.
- Heightened Sense Perception
- More Restful Sleep/Vivid Dreams
- Happier Attitude
- Increased Weight Loss
- Enhanced Physique, Stamina

While most of the above are obvious, some need more discussion.

Pain, for example, can affect many parts of the body. While injuries, obesity, poor posture, and other conditions can lead to pain, an often overlooked source of aches and pains is inflammation from toxins. Joint pain and Rheumatoid Arthritis are associated with toxin buildup in the joints, and chronic pain may also have toxin origins.

Fibromyalgia is a term used to describe a constellation of symptoms with no known cause. Many physicians deem fibromyalgia a psychosomatic problem—"all in your head." But the symptoms of fibromyalgia, such as fatigue, brain fog, mood disturbances, numbness and tingling in the extremities, and poor quality sleep are also very similar to Chronic Fatigue Syndrome (CFS), another condition with "unknown" causes. *Untaught*, more likely.

Research[98, 99, 100] has revealed that toxins play a large role in the onset of these two conditions, and our sauna detoxification protocol has provided relief to many who suffer these afflictions.

Peace of Mind

Past clients and patients have reported a sense of relief from worrying about contracting a serious medical condition once they have completed this protocol. The peace of mind that comes from understanding the two main factors of disease—poor nutrition and fat-stored toxins—and handling them both is priceless to them.

Are you considering pregnancy? Chemicals and heavy metals pass through the placenta to the fetus, which can lead to endocrine disorders, immune suppression, birth defects, and even miscarriage!

High concentrations of pesticide residues and heavy metals, especially mercury and lead, are found in mothers' breast milk and fed to nursing babies. Lowered IQ, lowered cognitive function, and mental retardation are linked to these xenobiotics.

Detoxination can reduce your own body burden to give you better peace of mind for a healthier baby. It is best for both partners to undergo the protocol several months before conception.

---

[98] Racciatti, Delia, Jacopo Vecchiet, Annalisa Ceccomancini, Francesco Ricci, and Eligio Pizzigallo. "Chronic fatigue syndrome following a toxic exposure." *Science of The Total Environment* 270, no. 1-3 (2001), 27-31. https://www.ncbi.nlm.nih.gov/pubmed/11327394.

[99] Vojdani, Aristo, and Charles W. Lapp. "The Relationship Between Chronic Fatigue Syndrome and Chemical Exposure." *Journal of Chronic Fatigue Syndrome* 5, no. 3-4 (1999), 207-221. https://doi.org/10.1300/J092v05n03_18.

[100] Ziem, Grace, and James McTamney. "Profile of Patients with Chemical Injury and Sensitivity." *Environmental Health Perspectives* 105 (1997), 417. https://www.ncbi.nlm.nih.gov/pmc/articles/PMC1469804/.

Keeping Up With the Millennials

Speaking of babies, Boomers are competing more and more with the Millennials for jobs. With a tough housing market, lingering effects of the recession, and less in retirement accounts due to interest rates, Baby Boomers have no guarantee that they can afford to retire at 65.

If you find yourself needing to have more vitality, stamina, cognitive function, and better rest at night to compete with the younger generations, then Detoxination may be right for you!

Drug Testing / Addiction / Rehabilitation

Those who are still craving drugs, even after being in a drug rehab program or quitting "cold turkey" will benefit from reducing the chemical residues that have accumulated in the tissues. Dr. Nenah Sylver states in her book *The Holistic Handbook of Sauna Therapy*, "Dr. Root observes that a significant 72% to 75% of the participants [of the Hubbard Protocol] remain drug-free, as evidenced by follow-up reports over a period of five years."

And chronic pot users needing to pass a drug screen can substantially reduce the time needed to clear trace amounts of THC from the body with this protocol. A chronic user may take up to 75 days to pass a drug screen; however, some can pass in just 10 days after our protocol.

Discussion

The bottom line benefits of Detoxination are your overall improved quality of life and health. Detoxination is the best preventive health measure you can do for yourself, *and your loved ones!*

We have found this protocol to be an effective anti-aging formula because it addresses the primary factors that produce the negative aspects to aging: the lifetime of toxin buildup in your body, toxic choices (i.e. smoking, drugs, excessive alcohol consumption), poor diet (processed "food products" and fast food, etc.), lack of exercise, and even medications.[101]

Energy levels and vitality are boosted, the so-called "Low T" (low testosterone in men) condition is reversed, stamina and strength are increased, and all cognitive processes—including memory, attention, focus, and coordination—are vastly improved.

On average, we have seen I.Q. scores increase 7 points after the protocol. Also, many people report that food tastes better, their vision is clearer, colors are brighter, and their skin is softer and younger looking. Even body odor is greatly improved.

By far, the most exciting benefit from Detoxination is the increased ability to lose weight once the toxins have been removed from the fat cells. Remember that the toxins were sequestered in the fat to protect the vital organs.

Some toxic endocrine-disrupting chemicals have been shown to be *obesogens* (foreign chemical compounds that disrupt normal development and balance of lipid metabolism, which in some cases, can lead to obesity.)

Obesogens are believed to work in several ways. They may change how a person's fat cells develop, meaning they may increase fat storage capacity or the number of fat cells.

---

[101] Antell, Darrick E., and Eva M. Taczanowski. "How Environment and Lifestyle Choices Influence the Aging Process." *Annals of Plastic Surgery* 43, no. 6 (1999), 585-588. https://www.ncbi.nlm.nih.gov/pubmed/10597816.

Also, obesogens may make it more difficult to maintain a healthy weight, by changing how the body regulates feelings of hunger and fullness, or increasing the effects of high fat and high sugar diets.[102]

To help your body burn the excess fat, you must force the toxins from those fat cells and get them out of the body safely and effectively. Detoxination can do just that!

I must disclose, however, that your results may vary. There are too many variables affecting outcomes, but we strongly believe that this protocol is the most significant way to positively change your life.

When you can perform better in all aspects of your life because of your excellent health, you become wealthier than what possessions and money can offer. You have more freedom, happiness, and better potential to increase your financial condition!

---

[102] "Obesogens." National Institute of Environmental Health Sciences. https://www.niehs.nih.gov/health/topics/conditions/obesity/obesogens/index.cfm.

Summary of Benefits Presented to the EPA

I will conclude the discussion of benefits with the following Table 2.2 compiled from the results of 120 individuals treated using the Hubbard Method. These results were presented by my father and a team from FASE in May, 1985, at the *Proceedings of the National Conference on Hazardous Wastes and Environmental Emergencies* held in Cincinnati, Ohio.[4]

Table 2.2

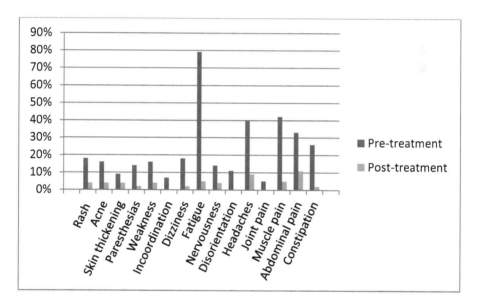

From this chart you can see that fatigue was reported by 78% of the study participants, and it is a frequent complaint of all chemical exposure cases my father has treated. These post-treatment findings are common with sauna detoxification.

While the Hubbard Method provided a valuable foundation of knowledge and experience, we have learned a great deal since 1982 and no longer strictly follow the original protocol. Detoxination is the culmination of all our experience, as well as advancements in research and technology.

Key improvements of our ***Get Detoxinated!***™ program include:

- Timing niacin intake for improved efficacy
- Use of full spectrum infrared sauna to increase toxicant output is less time
- Use of binders to capture and expel toxins from GI tract
- Reduction in overall time commitment
- Expanded coaching on nutrition and toxin avoidance

CHAPTER 3
The Detoxination Protocol

Before we take a deep-dive into the protocol, it is important that you know when Detoxination is contraindicated (conditions or circumstances that indicate that this protocol should not be done). Following are the main issues that need to be discussed so you can make an informed decision whether or not to proceed with Detoxination.

Contraindications / Preclusions / Advice

Detoxination is not for everyone, although everyone needs it! If you have any of the following conditions, we recommend our medically supervised Detoxination at one of our Centers, careful consideration, or not even doing it.

Do not attempt to self-treat any disease with infrared sauna without direct supervision by a licensed health care provider. Be sure to verify with your primary care physician if sauna is appropriate for you (We have prepared a Treatment Information and Sign-off form that you may download at https://www.GetDetoxinated.com/book/ to provide your health practitioner).

Adrenal Fatigue Syndrome

Those in early AFS (stages 1 and 2) generally can tolerate sauna heat well. Those with advanced AFS, on the other hand, are usually quite fragile and sauna may make the condition worse.

Start at 50 mg niacin and only increment 50-100 mg when your previous dose no longer causes a flush. Begin your program with 15 minutes of lower temperature sauna (110°-120°F) for the first few days. Try sitting in the sauna as it heats up. If, after the first few days, you feel you can increase your time, then do so. After the first week, try increasing the temperature as well. Also, stay hydrated and replace your electrolytes appropriately.

Alcohol / Alcohol Abuse

Excess alcohol consumption can cause dehydration. Alcohol decreases the body's production of anti-diuretic hormone, which is used by the body to reabsorb water. With less anti-diuretic hormone available, your body loses more fluid than normal through increased urination.

Breastfeeding

Lactating mothers cannot participate in the program for the same reason. For the mother, breast milk has been shown to be an effective means of reducing her body burden of toxic materials. Studies have shown that breast milk tends to contain high concentrations of toxins.

Cardiovascular Conditions

Individuals with cardiovascular conditions (high or low blood pressure, irregular heartbeat, congestive heart failure, or impaired coronary circulation), or those who are taking medications that might affect blood pressure, should exercise extreme caution when exposed to prolonged heat.

Heat stress increases cardiac output and blood flow due to the body's effort to transfer internal body heat to the outside environment via the skin (perspiration) and respiratory system. This takes place primarily due to major changes in the heart rate, which has the potential to increase by 30 beats per minute for each degree of increase in core body temperature.

Children

The core body temperature rises much faster in children than adults. This occurs due to a higher metabolic rate per body mass, limited circulatory adaptation to increased cardiac demands, and the inability to regulate body temperature by sweating. Children age 4 and up, who take instruction well, are able to undergo Detoxination when accompanied by an adult.

Chronic Conditions / Diseases Associated with a Reduced Ability to Perspire

Parkinson's disease, Multiple Sclerosis, central nervous system tumors, and Diabetes with neuropathy are conditions that are associated with impaired sweating. Consult with your physician before attempting Detoxination.

The Elderly

The ability to maintain core body temperature decreases with age. This is primarily due to circulatory conditions and decreased sweat gland function. The body must be able to activate its natural cooling processes in order to maintain core body temperature.

Fever

An individual who has a fever should not use a sauna. Although the underlying cause of the fever (viruses or bacteria) cannot survive the high heat, fever is a stress to the body's regulatory system. Dehydration and a weakened immune system will only be exacerbated by sauna heat.

Heat Sensitivity

An individual who has heat sensitivity should consider not using a sauna.

Hemophiliacs / Individuals Prone to Bleeding

The use of sauna should be avoided by anyone who is predisposed to bleeding.

Hypothyroidism

A characteristic of hypothyroidism is the decreased ability to sweat or not sweat at all. Sauna can improve thyroid function and the ability to sweat. Start with shorter sauna sessions at lower temperatures and then slowly increase both time and heat each with each successive session.

Implants (Infrared Sauna Notice)

Metal pins, rods, artificial joints, or any other surgical implants generally reflect infrared waves and thus are not heated by infrared waves. Nevertheless, you should consult your surgeon prior to using an infrared sauna.

Certainly the use of an infrared sauna must be discontinued if you experience pain near any such implants. Silicone does absorb infrared energy. Implanted silicone or silicone prostheses for nose or ear replacement may be warmed by the infrared waves. Because silicone melts at over 200°C (392°F), it should not be adversely affected by the usage of an infrared sauna. It is still advised that you check with your surgeon, and possibly a representative from the implant manufacturer, to be certain.

Joint Injury/Pain

Recent acute joint injuries should not be heated for the first 48 hours or until the hot and swollen symptoms subside. If you have a joint or joints that are chronically hot and swollen, these joints may respond poorly to vigorous heating of any kind.

Joint pain, on the other hand, benefits greatly from sauna heat, and many report that their chronic joint pain is permanently relieved after completing the protocol.

Medications

Individuals who are using prescription drugs should seek the advice of their prescribing physician or a pharmacist for possible changes in the drugs' effects when the body is exposed to infrared waves or elevated body temperature. Diuretics, barbiturates, and beta-blockers may impair the body's natural heat loss mechanisms. Some over-the-counter drugs such as antihistamines may also cause the body to be more prone to heat stroke. Medications delivered through a dermal patch may be affected by heat.

Be aware that, our Detoxination protocols draw any fat soluble drugs out of the fat cells into the bloodstream which can lead to severe withdrawal conditions.

Menstruation

Heating of the lower back area of women during their menstrual period may temporarily increase the menstrual flow. Some women endure this process to gain the pain relief commonly associated with their cycle, whereas others simply choose to avoid sauna use during that time of the month.

Pacemaker/Defibrillator (Infrared Sauna Notice)

Any magnets used in the construction of an infrared sauna unit may interfere with the output of pacemakers. Please discuss the possible risks this may cause with your physician.

Pregnancy

Since it would be very dangerous for the developing fetus to be exposed to the higher blood levels of toxic materials that are released into the mother's circulation by this program, Detoxination cannot be allowed during pregnancy.

Preparation

As you begin your journey into our life-changing Detoxination Protocol, you will need to do a bit of preparation. Three key areas will impact your successful completion: Mindset, Body Prep, and Equipment.

Mindset

"The secret of change is to focus all of your energy, not on fighting the old, but on building the new." Socrates

Detoxination requires a shift in mindset and a better awareness of the threats that our lifestyle choices may present to our health, vitality, and longevity. Your success will be achieved by implementing these small changes in your daily life, especially during the Protocol. Remember, it's taken a lifetime to become toxic, so now commit to just two weeks of needed Detoxination.

Believe it or not, the toughest aspect of Detoxination is *mindset*. You have to be willing to take a hard look at your daily routine, choices, and even the people with whom you associate. You get both good things and bad from these three categories, so let's get a handle on the bad things.

DAILY ROUTINE

We are all creatures of habit, so when we get up we follow a routine. After the obligatory toilet stop, we may wash our hair in the shower or bath, brush our teeth, do our makeup or shave our whiskers, put on antiperspirant, and fix our hair. Or something along these lines.

According to the Huffington Post, the average woman puts 515 synthetic chemicals on her body every day without knowing it.[103] Men average around 85 chemicals. Most of these products are applied directly to the largest organ of the body: the skin. A whopping 60 percent of these chemicals are absorbed through the skin and into our bodies where they bioaccumulate in the dermis layers and lead to inflammation.

Antiperspirant contains high levels of aluminum, and toothpaste contains fluoride, both of which are extremely neurotoxic. And these tend to be the only two ingredients we can pronounce on the product labels!

Your routine could also take you to a fast food joint for a quick breakfast, or popping a prepackaged "food" product into the microwave before heading out the door. What you wind up with has little to no nutritional value (other than the synthetically fortified variety). Worse, it contains a lot of artificial flavors, food colors, preservatives, MSG, and more unpronounceable chemicals that poison your body.

Remember, if you can't pronounce an ingredient, then it is probably not good for you. Also, the flavor enhancer known as Monosodium Glutamic Acid, or MSG, goes by many names such as Soy Protein, Textured Protein, and anything "hydrolyzed." However, no matter how it appears, it is still linked to a host of health issues including fibromyalgia, obesity, fatty liver, high insulin and blood sugar, high cholesterol, metabolic syndrome, high blood pressure, disturbances

[103] "The Average Woman Puts 515 Synthetic Chemicals On Her Body Every Day." HuffPost. Last modified March 7, 2016. https://www.huffpost.com/entry/synthetic-chemicals-skincare_n_56d8ad09e4b0000de403d995.

in the gut-brain connection, neurological and brain health issues, and much more.[104]

CHOICES

You may have already noticed that your daily routine involves products purchased as a result of choices you made earlier. Your daily routine and the choices you make synergistically set you up for failure on a program like Detoxination. Therefore, you really need to be prepared to rethink your choices before you start. You can replace the toxic versions of most products with chemical-free and organic ones. It may not be easy to discard your old products all at once, so work them out of your life over a little bit at a time.

Later in this book we share ideas on products we use or make ourselves to live a more chemical-free life.

The most important choice to reassess is food. Always strive to make great choices with food. We have already discussed the pitfalls of GMOs and preprocessed, packaged food products, so let's change our mindset on organic fruits and vegetables. What's the number one argument against organic? That's right, *cost*!

Remember at the beginning of this book I revealed that the average American family of four will spend on health care upwards of $28,166 per year? Just think how much tasty, nutritious, organic food could have been purchased with that kind of money! And you would be healthier!

You'll also find as you give up the chips, cookies, pastries, and other garbage snacks, that the organic food budget magically grows. But

---

[104] Dobbins, Robin. *Seemingly Sound Eating yet Severe Bodily Damage: Inflammation Is Silently Assassinating You*. Bloomington, IN: AuthorHouse, 2015.

don't worry about your cravings for all that sugar, Detoxination will help you get past those.

While you're at it, stop with the sodas! Especially diet sodas. I find it fascinating that manufacturers can still legally call them "diet" simply because they contain less sugar. The artificial sweeteners are far more toxic and actually *cause* obesity[105] as well as type 2 diabetes[106]!

Nutrition is about the right vitamins and minerals for your body, so stop looking for that magic, one-size-fits-all diet! There is one diet, however, that should be discussed for its potentially synergistic detox qualities, the Ketogenic Diet.

Many of you reading this book will have already heard of, or are currently on, a Ketogenic Diet. This eating plan is all about minimizing your carbs and upping your fats to get your body to use fat as a form of energy. While everyone's body and intake needs are slightly different, that typically translates to: 60 to 75 percent of your calories from fat, 15 to 30 percent of your calories from protein, and 5 to 10 percent of your calories from carbs.

After about two to seven days of this eating routine, you go into something called ketosis, or the state your body enters when it doesn't have enough carbs for your cells to use for energy. Then it starts making *ketones*, or organic compounds that your body then uses in place of those missing carbs, while burning fat for more energy. Although we are in favor of Keto for a period of 30-60 days prior to and during this Protocol we do not recommend it for the long

---

[105] Gain weight by "going diet?" Artificial sweeteners and the neurobiology of sugar cravings: Neuroscience 2010. *Yale J Biol Med*. 2010;83(2):101-8. https://www.ncbi.nlm.nih.gov/pmc/articles/PMC2892765/

[106] Strawbridge, Holly. "Artificial Sweeteners: Sugar-free, but at What Cost?" *Harvard Health Blog*. January 8, 2018. https://www.health.harvard.edu/blog/artificial-sweeteners-sugar-free-but-at-what-cost-201207165030.

run. Not all the required vitamins and minerals are available on a strict ketogenic diet.

If you really want to identify what is the best diet for you and for weight loss, we recommend you read *The Metabolic Typing Diet* by William Wolcott and Trish Fahey.

Another important choice you should make is the kind of water you put into your body. Proper hydration is essential while on the Detoxination Protocol, and you only want to drink the best water. We will cover this topic in greater detail on page 161 of Chapter 4.

PEOPLE

Your mindset is all that matters, but the people you surround yourself with may not be as supportive as you'd like. They will likely have a different mindset about Detoxination, and they may try to lure you into activities that will be counterproductive to your goals. Some of your associates may need to be completely shut out of your personal life temporarily while you complete your protocol. It's just the way it is.

Most people are completely oblivious or apathetic to the toxin problem. The new choices you make may cause them to mock and tease you, but don't be put off by it. Stay firm in your resolve to carry on with your Detoxination Protocol. Maybe someday they will take notice of the awesome changes they see in you—like your skin tone, your bright eyes, your well-rested look in the morning, your stamina, your weight loss, and how much better you seem to think!

Body Prep

Before you tackle our 2-week Detoxination Protocol, you should work on the health and proper functioning of your detox organs: the liver, kidneys, and colon.

I often recommend our patients and wellness clients to acquire, read, and follow the sage advice from Dr. Joseph Pizzorno in his book, *The Toxin Solution*. Dr. Pizzorno's mentors said years ago that death begins in the colon! The wrong kind of bacteria in your gut produces toxins that damage physiology, so the first step is healing the gut.

He touches on how to kill the bad bacteria with goldenseal while leaving the good bacteria alone. His favorite food-as-medicine to heal the gut is cabbage juice, which is very high in glutamine.

After working on the gut, clean up the liver because the biggest source of toxins afflicting the liver is an unhealthy gut. By taking enough B vitamins and iron along with herbs like dandelion, the liver gets the support it needs.

The third part of the Body Prep is the kidneys. Years ago, renal failure was unusual; today, there is an abundance of dialysis centers, and Dr. Pizzorno attributes this to the toxic load that has overwhelmed the kidneys. Most damage to the kidneys comes from reduced blood supply coming to them. Dr. Pizzorno recommends using beet juice because it's so high in the amino acid arginine, which helps dilate blood vessels to the kidneys.

Blueberries (and blueberry juice) are another superfood for the kidneys. They contain antioxidants called anthocyanidins, which decrease inflammation in blood vessels going to the kidneys, thus allowing for more blood flow.

These nutrients improve how well the kidneys cleanse themselves. Pizzorno's protocols are extremely worth doing before ours.

AMALGAM FILLINGS

Mercury dental fillings (also called silver fillings), or amalgams, have been in use for more than 150 years, despite the fact that mercury is one of the most potent neurotoxins known to medical science. Dental amalgam is an antiquated filling material that's typically a mixture of 50 percent mercury and 50 percent other metals like copper, tin, silver and zinc.

Mercury is continuously released from amalgam fillings. It is absorbed and retained in the body, particularly in the brain, kidneys, liver, lungs, and gastrointestinal tract. The output of mercury is intensified by the number of fillings and other activities, such as chewing, teeth-grinding, and the consumption of hot liquids.

According to Dr. Joseph Mercola, amalgam fillings can release an average of 10 micrograms of mercury vapor into your mouth every day. Studies have suggested that dental amalgam is responsible for at least 60-95 percent of mercury in human tissues.[107]

The target organ of mercury is the brain. Unfortunately, mercury toxicity is not often included in the differential diagnosis of common subjective complaints such as fatigue, anxiety, depression, odd paresthesias, memory loss, and difficulty concentrating.[108]

Mercury is so toxic that if the amount of mercury contained in an old thermometer is dumped in a small lake, that lake would be closed off as an environmental hazard. Yet more mercury than that is put into a single amalgam filling!

A better alternative is to have amalgams replaced with composite fillings by a biological dentist who is trained in safe amalgam removal. Request they use BPA- and fluoride-free materials, as well.

---

[107] "There Is NO Safe Level of Using Mercury Dental Fillings (Amalgam)." Mercola.com. Last modified May 9, 2015. https://articles.mercola.com/sites/articles/archive/2015/05/09/mercury-dental-fillings.aspx.

[108] Mercury toxicity and treatment: a review of the literature. *J Environ Public Health*. 2011. https://www.ncbi.nlm.nih.gov/pmc/articles/PMC3253456/.

PRIMARY CARE PHYSICIAN REVIEW AND PHYSICAL EXAM

It is strongly recommended that you discuss this protocol with your primary health care professional and even get a physical exam before beginning our Detoxination program. You can download an overview to present to your health care professional that explains the protocol sufficiently to make an informed recommendation. This form may be found at: https://www.GetDetoxinated.com/forms/.

TESTING FOR CHEMICALS/HEAVY METALS

While not required, test kits may be ordered from labs such as Great Plains Laboratories or Doctor's Data, to test your blood, urine, hair, and even feces if you so desire. We offer these, as well as instant drug screens (which may be purchased from Amazon), to our clients and patients before Detoxination, and 30 days after.

Note that blood tests tend to reflect higher "after" readings due to the newly mobilized toxins still circulating through the body. This is why it is best to continue with binders after completing the program and waiting 30 days before re-testing.

Equipment and Supplies

Following is a list of the equipment, tools, consumables, and other accessories you may need to complete Detoxination. Most of these items can be purchased from our website (see below):

- Sauna (infrared preferred)
- Aerobic exercise equipment (i.e. exercycle, treadmill, rebounder, and/or elliptical machine) or space for jogging
- Resistance bands (optional)

Tools/Meters/Scales/Measuring Devices

- Weight scale for "Before" and "After" sauna cycles
- Measuring scale for powdered products
- Thermometer (optional)
- Downloadable forms (optional) which are found at https://www.GetDetoxinated.com/book/
- Blood Pressure Cuff (optional)
- BMI/Fat % meter (optional)
- 100% pure, organic cranberry juice (for flavoring of oils and Cal-Mag beverage discussed later)
- Measuring spoons (½ teaspoon, teaspoon and tablespoon)
- Electric kettle for quickly boiling water for Cal-Mag (optional but very handy!)
- Lidded carafe (hot/cold preferred)
- Dixie cups for electrolytes and oils (recommended)
- Glass drinking bottle or stainless steel canister for filtered water in the sauna. No plastic bottles!
- Towels (hand towel for wiping off sweat and bath towel)
- Protective pads (recommended/discussed later)
- Aqua shoes or workout shoes for exercise and protection

Supplements and Binders

The following list of vitamins, minerals, and electrolytes are the recommended values and quantities for a 30-day protocol. Niacin is available in capsule or powder form. Niacin capsules are included in this list in three levels for convenience. In our Centers, we manually measure niacin doses obtained from the bulk powder form.

- Vitamin A & D 10,000 IU & 400 IU - 100 Softgels - Active Ingredients: Vitamin A (from fish liver oil) 10,000 IU, Vitamin D (from fish liver oil) 400 IU
- Vitamin E 400 IU - 150 Softgels - Active Ingredients: Vitamin E (as d-alpha tocopherol from soy) 400 IU
- Evening Primrose Oil 500 mg - 100 Softgels - Active Ingredients: Evening Primrose Seed Oil 500 mg Gamma Linolenic Acid GLA – 45 mg
- Vitamin B-1 100 mg - 50 Capsules - Active Ingredients: Thiamine (vitamin B-1) (as Thiamine mononitrate)
- Vitamin B1 250 mg - 100 Capsules - Active Ingredients: Thiamine (vitamin B-1) (as Thiamine Mononitrate) 250 mg
- Niacin 100 mg - 100 Capsules - Active Ingredients: Niacin (as Nicotinic Acid) 100 mg
- Niacin 500 mg. - 60 Capsules - Active Ingredients: Niacin (as Nicotinic Acid) 500 mg
- Niacin 1,000 mg. - 75 Capsules - Active Ingredients: Niacin (as Nicotinic Acid) 1,000 mg
- B-50 Complex - 150 Capsules - Active Ingredients: Vitamin B1 (as Thiamine HCI) 50 mg Vitamin B-2 (as riboflavin) 50 mg, Vitamin B-6 (as pyridoxine HCI) 50 mg, Vitamin B-12 (as cyanocobalamin) 50 mcg, Folic Acid (as Folate) 50 mcg, Biotin (as d-Biotin) 50 mcg, Pantothenic Acid (as

calcium D-Pantothenate) 50 mg Other Ingredients: Gelatin,
cellulose, silicon dioxide, and magnesium stearate.

- Vitamin C 1,000 mg - 100 Capsules - Active Ingredients:
  Vitamin C (as ascorbic acid) 1,000 mg
- Calcium Gluconate 9% - 16 oz. Powder - Active Ingredients:
  Calcium (as Calcium Gluconate 9%) 900 mg
- DNA-Negative Soy Lecithin - 16 oz. Granules - Active
  Ingredients: Soy Lecithin Granules one scoop 6.5 grams
- Magnesium Carbonate 29% - 2 oz. Powder - Active
  Ingredients: Magnesium (as Magnesium Carbonate 29%)
  185 mg
- Multi Mineral - 200 Tablets - Active Ingredients: Calcium
  (as Calcium Carbonate) 500 mg, Iron (as Ferrous Fumarate)
  18 mg, Magnesium (as Magnesium Oxide) 250 mg,
  Manganese (as Manganese Citrate) 4 mg, Zinc (as Zinc
  Citrate) 15 mg, Potassium (as Potassium Carbonate Iodide)
  45 mg, Copper (as Copper Gluconate) 2 mg, Chromium (as
  Chromium Polynicotinate) 120 mcg, Iodine (as Potassium
  Iodide) 225 mcg, Selenium (as L-Selenomethionine) 70
  mcg, Molybdenum (as Sodium Molybdate) 75 mcg, Cobalt
  (as Cyanocobalamin) 2 mcg
- Cell Salts (aka Plasma Electrolytes) - 4 oz. Tablets - Active
  Ingredients: Calcium (as Calcium sulfate, dicalcium
  phosphate) 0.3 mg, Iron (as Ferric Orthophospate) .1 mg,
  Phosphorus (as Magnesium Phosphate, Ferric
  Orthophosphate, Dicalcium Phosphate, Potassium
  Phosphate) .3 mg, Magnesium (as Magnesium Phosphate)
  .1 mg, Chloride (as Potassium Chloride, Sodium Chloride) .1
  mg, Silica (as Silicon Dioxide), Potassium (as Potassium
  Chloride Potassium Sulfate, Potassium Phosphate) 2 mg
- Potassium 99mg - 125 Tablets - Active Ingredients:
  Potassium (as Potassium Gluconate) 99 mg

- Salt tablet - 200 Tablets - Active Ingredients: Chloride (as Sodium Chloride) 300 mg, Sodium (as Sodium Chloride) 190 mg
- Organic Apple Cider Vinegar for Cal-Mag
- Polyunsaturated cold pressed oils (i.e. organic flax seed oil, hemp oil, sunflower oil, and walnut oil are good examples)
- Food grade Calcium Bentonite or Micronized Zeolite Clay
- Activated Charcoal (AC)
- Cholestepure (optional binder/discussed later)
- Nascent or Lugol's Iodine (optional, recommended)

Most of these recommended products are available for purchase from our online store at https://www.GetDetoxinated.com/shop/. Register to receive discounts on products and notices of specials.

Step-By-Step Detoxination Protocol

WARNING: Do not attempt this protocol without a thorough understanding of all aspects and procedures. Supervision during the protocol is recommended due to risks of heat exhaustion, dehydration, and drug residue manifestations. An observer may be a detox partner, a family member, or associate with whom you can keep in constant communication by text or checkup call.

This protocol has been shown to balance the mobilization of toxins with the elimination of toxins when followed correctly. It is inadvisable to interrupt the protocol for any reason. Once you commence the protocol, mobilized toxins must be allowed to safely exit your body. Xenobiotics that have not been eliminated via sweat or captured with binders will eventually undergo multiple entero-hepatic recirculation cycles. The potential acute toxicity from the high volume of these once-sequestered poisons may overwhelm your liver or kidneys. To prevent unwanted liver or renal damage, avoid skipping any days and avoid shortcuts to the protocol unless the word "optional" is stated.

Mobilized xenobiotics may cause headaches, nausea, dizziness, fatigue, or other unwanted symptoms. These will pass if you push on through the protocol as instructed. Stay well hydrated and replenish electrolytes after each sauna cycle.

While a 2-week protocol can be very effective in reducing your toxic body burden, longer programs of around 30 days are preferred.

The *Get Detoxinated!*™ Program

We encourage you to participate in the *Get Detoxinated!* Program by recording your Detoxination experience on downloadable worksheets. Upon completion of your Detoxination, please fax, email, or send by mail copies of your completed worksheets to:

Detoxination Wellness Centers
2706 Mercantile Drive
Rancho Cordova, CA 95742

We will review and add them to our research database. These are completely anonymous if you wish, and our research program is optional. Even if you decide not to participate, the forms and instructions found at https://www.GetDetoxinated.com/book/ will help you monitor your own progress during the program.

By submitting your logs and information, you consent to our unrestricted use of the data to track statistics, such as niacin doses and correlated manifestations, sauna durations, supplementation, blood pressures, results, and other factors.

This is not a formal research study. Your name will never be used without your written consent.

Participation in this program is voluntary. If, at any time and for any reason, you would prefer not to participate in this program, please feel free not to. If at any time you would like to stop participating, please tell us. You may withdraw from this program at any time, and you will not be penalized in any way for deciding to end your participation.

If you decide to withdraw from this program, please contact us if you do not want data collected from you to be used.

Detoxination Protocol Preparation

Niacin

First calculate your Target Niacin Dose (TND) of 10mg/kg. To convert pounds to kilograms, simply divide your weight in pounds by 2.205. Your TND will be 10 times that number (example found on page 125).

Your first goal is to reach your TND for the ideal rebound lipolysis state (as illustrated in Fig. 2.4 on page 71). Once you reach that level—usually within 10 days—continue increasing at tolerable increments daily until you reach either the End Phenomenon, as described on page 74, or 14 days minimum.

With niacin, it is best to start at 50-100 mg. A red skin flush (usually accompanied by an itchy, prickly sensation) is a great indicator that you are taking enough niacin. The flush should dissipate after 45 minutes, on average. No flushing or less flushing than the previous day means you should increase your niacin dose. Incrementally increase the daily dose by 100-200 mg, as needed. If you find you cannot tolerate the current level, do that same level (or slightly less) the next day. Within a short period, such as a day or two, you should be able to tolerate the next increase.

Food can help to slow the negative flushing effects and possible nausea caused by niacin, but the desired rebound lipolysis will be slower to "trigger" as well. Similarly, while being digested the pill form of niacin will take longer to trigger rebound lipolysis over the powdered form.

Don't overdo the niacin increases, but if you find you can easily tolerate the 100 mg increases, try 200 mg on the next day. We have found that 300 mg daily increases are very doable with individuals who weigh 170 lb. or more.

The average niacin level achieved while on this program is 1,800 mg (1.8 g); however, some will get as high as 3,000 mg (3 g) during a 14-day protocol. On a 30-day program, do not exceed 5 g without the express consent of your primary care practitioner.

The use of any aspirin, NSAIDs, or steroids will have a blocking effect on the niacin flush. Avoid taking these medications while on the Program.

Cautionary Note:

The use of niacin during Detoxination may produce many side-effects that you may find uncomfortable. Both niacin and mobilized toxins circulating your body are responsible for these conditions. Discontinue niacin if you cannot push through these symptoms:
- Skin flushing, redness, tingling, irritation, and itching
- Dizziness and sometimes confusion
- Rapid and/or irregular heartbeat
- Nausea
- Vomiting
- Abdominal pain
- Diarrhea
- Difficulty breathing, shortness of breath
- Rapid heartbeat (tachycardia)
- Severe hypotension (discontinue Detoxination)
- Insomnia (lack of sleep)
- Cramping and/or pain in the leg muscles (drink Cal-Mag)
- Sensation of being chilled and/or sweating
- Lightheadedness and dizziness
- Symptoms similar to flu

Note: Taking 1-2 aspirin (325 mg) can provide needed relief from these symptoms.

Sample Niacin Dosing Schedule

Example:

Weight is 180 lb.

180 / 2.205 = 81.63 kg

81.63 X 10 = 816.3 mg

TND = **816.3 mg**

The table on the right shows the number of days to reach the TND (or next highest dose) based on a tolerated schedule.

	Suggested Niacin Schedules		
Day	Light	Moderate	Aggressive
1	50	100	100
2	100	300	300
3	200	500	600
4	300	700	**900**
5	400	**900**	1100
6	500	1000	1300
7	600	1100	1500
8	700	1200	1700
9	800	1300	1900
10	**900**	1400	2100
11	1000	1500	2300
12	1100	1600	2500
13	1200	1700	2700
14	1300	1800	2900

Begin your daily session by measuring the current niacin dose. For powder, it is best place a Dixie cup, or similar container, on a gram scale then "zero-out" the weight of the container with the tare button. Using the ½ teaspoon measuring spoon, scoop the powdered niacin into the cup until reaching the desired dose.

Add at least 2 ounces of water and mix thoroughly. To improve the taste, add a tablespoon of 100% organic cranberry juice.

Niacin in pill form can be dosed by dividing the current dose by the pill strength of the niacin to arrive at the quantity of pills required.

Consume your niacin dose two hours prior to your session. During the waiting period you can finish preparing for the daily session.

Cal-Mag Recipe

Make a fresh batch of Cal-Mag, if needed (one batch may last up to 3 days when covered and properly refrigerated):

1. Boil a cup of water
2. Mix into a large (1 liter min.) heat resistant, lidded container:
   1 level tablespoon calcium gluconate powder
   ½ teaspoon magnesium carbonate powder
   1.5 tablespoons of apple cider vinegar
3. Stir/shake very well to thoroughly combine all ingredients
4. Let sit for approximately three minutes
5. Add cup of hot water, stir/shake, and let sit for a few minutes
6. Add cup of cold/ice water and stir
7. Pour into a glass
8. Stir in 2 oz. of 100% organic cranberry juice to flavor
9. Cover and refrigerate remainder for the next session

Notes:

This mixture makes 1 - 2 days' worth of Cal-Mag.

Apple cider vinegar (ACV) is an activator for a necessary chemical reaction to balance the pH of the calcium and magnesium (calcium needs an acidic base in which to release positive ions for interaction with cellular structures, but magnesium is alkaline). Apple cider vinegar allows the calcium and magnesium to be absorbed into body tissue. Without it, the calcium would just run right through you.

It also gives you a great dose of potassium to balance sodium, regulate water retention, and balance blood pressure. This can work to eliminate migraine headaches and other serious aches and pains.

The cranberry juice improves the taste of the Cal-Mag mixture.

Electrolytes

Prepare electrolytes for every 30 minutes of sauna time as follows:

Place in a Dixie cup, or similar container:

- 4 Cell salt pills
- 1 Potassium
- 1 Sodium chloride (salt) pill

These will be consumed immediately upon exiting the sauna or if you feel headachy, nauseated, dizzy, or weak during your sauna session (symptoms associated with electrolyte imbalance, dehydration, and/or heat exhaustion).

Vitamin and Mineral Schedule

This is also the best time to prepare the vitamins and minerals you will take after your daily session.

The following table shows proportionate vitamin and mineral increases at various levels of niacin doses. Note: niacin doses up to 5,000 mg (5 g) are attained in the 30-day program. If you have not reached the "End Phenomenon" after 14 days then continue the protocol, if desired.

Remember these are "replenishments" for vitamins and minerals lost to sweat, on average, during a Detoxination session. Even if you are regularly supplementing your diet with vitamins and minerals, these doses are recommended to bring your body back into balance.

Vitamin Table

Compare your current niacin dose to the ranges in the outlined box to determine which level corresponds to the vitamin range you need.

	Level 1	Level 2	Level 3	Level 4	Level 5
Niacin	**100 to 400 mg**	**500 to 1,400 mg**	**1,500 to 2,400 mg**	**2,500 to 3,400 mg**	**3,500 to 5,000 mg**
Vitamin A	5,000 to 10,000 IU	20,000 IU	30,000 IU	50,000 IU	50,000 IU
Vitamin B complex	2 tablets	3 tablets	4 tablets	5 tablets	6 tablets
Vitamin B1	350 to 600 mg	400 to 650 mg	450 to 700 mg	750 to 1,250 mg	800 to 1,300 mg
Vitamin C	250 to 1,000 mg	2 to 3 g	3 to 4 g	4 to 5 g	5 to 6 g
Vitamin D	400 IU	800 IU	1,200 IU	2,000 IU	2,000 IU
Vitamin E	800 IU	1,200 IU	1,600 IU	2,000 IU	2,400 IU

Fat soluble vitamins such as A, D, and E need fatty acids for absorption, so pair foods that are rich in these nutrients (many vegetables are) with a source of healthy fat, like nuts or oil.

Mineral Table
(All values in mg)

These mineral doses follow the same niacin dose levels from the Vitamin Table. A good multi-mineral tablet may contain sufficient levels of these minerals to equate the level to the number of tablets required for the niacin level. For example, at niacin level 2, you would take 2 multi-mineral tablets.

	Level 1	Level 2	Level 3	Level 4	Level 5
Calcium	500 to 1,000	1,000 to 1,500	1,500 to 2,000	2,000 to 2,500	2,500 to 3,000
Magnesium	250 to 500	500 to 750	750 to 1,000	1,000 to 1,250	1,250 to 1,500
Iron	18-36	36-54	54-72	72-90	90-108
Zinc	15-30	30-45	45-60	60-75	75-90
Manganese	4-8	8-12	12-16	16-20	20-24
Copper	2-4	4-6	6-8	8-10	10-12
Potassium	45-90	90-135	135-180	180-225	225-270
Iodine	.225 to .450	.450 to .675	.675 to .900	.900 to 1.125	1.125 to 1.350

Vitamins and minerals synergistically work together, so take them around the same time—preferably soon after each session. Avoid taking vitamins at bedtime. Some vitamins will provide a boost of energy that may cause insomnia.

Binders and Oils

Four tablespoons of cold pressed polyunsaturated oils (organic flax seed, hemp, sunflower, etc.) are mixed in a cup with cranberry juice and consumed before exercising. The oils reduce reabsorption of mobilized toxins while providing another lipid with which some toxins will bind for excretion. Note that the oils tend to leak through Dixie cups after a short while.

Activated charcoal—not the type used for barbecuing—is a type of charcoal that's processed to make it more porous. It works by trapping toxins and chemicals in the gut and preventing their absorption. The charcoal's porous texture has a negative electrical charge, which causes it to attract positively charged molecules like toxins. This helps it bind xenobiotics in the gut. Because activated charcoal is not absorbed by your body, it can carry the bound toxins out of your body in feces.

As an alternative for those sensitive to edible oils, another option would be to combine AC with a plant sterol, such as Cholestepure from a company called Pure Encapsulations. Cholestepure is a substitute for the pharmaceutical cholestyramine, which may upset the stomach. When Cholestepure is combined with AC, it is ideal to have some fat in the digestive tract. Polyunsaturated, cold pressed oils or another source of dietary fat can help stimulate bile flow to aid the adsorption of toxins by the AC and Cholestepure.

At the conclusion of each daily session it is recommended to consume a tablespoon of Bentonite or micronized zeolite clay mixed with a cup of water to capture additional xenobiotics in the gut. Micronized zeolite has the added benefit of permeating into the bloodstream in order to adsorb toxins in blood before they can be deposited in the brain, bone, or adipose fat stores.

In severe toxicity situations headaches and nausea may occur during the night. It is helpful to take activated charcoal at bedtime in order to handle the xenobiotics still flowing through your system. Do not take activated charcoal within two hours of medications, as much of these drugs may be adsorbed before the body can utilize them.

Session Notes
Time of Day

The Detoxination Protocol is best done earlier in the day, but there are no hard and fast rules on when it should be undertaken. Keep in mind that vitamins and minerals are best replenished directly after your daily session, so evening sessions may provide an unwanted boost of energy at bedtime.

It is recommended to keep to a 24-hour schedule so you start around the same time each day. You are disrupting your body's normal cycles and rhythms with Detoxination, therefore, it is best to stay on a schedule to help the body adjust to these new activities.

Weighing In and Out

It is important to weigh yourself at the beginning of each session—with the clothing you will be wearing in the sauna—and then again after each session to determine whether or not you have hydrated yourself appropriately. The two weights should be closely matched. Otherwise, you need to drink more if your weight was less post-session. If you weigh more when you exit the sauna, then you consumed more than enough fluids during the session.

An adult male can easily sweat out 1-1.5 gallons of fluid in a full, medically supervised (4-5 hour) session in a dry sauna, and a person can sweat several quarts of fluid during a 2-hour FIR sauna session.

Sauna

Preheat your sauna at least 15 minutes prior to your session. The heat in infrared saunas is immediately available. However, the heat may not be to your liking until more of the sauna is warmed up. It is recommended to turn infrared saunas up to their maximum setting in order to prevent cycling of the infrared heating units.

Traditional convection saunas will require more time for the protocol. Plan 90-120 minutes of sauna at 15-20 minute intervals (with breaks) and 21-30 days for optimal results.

Protective Pads

We recommend covering the sauna seat and floor with a protective pad or towel. White is preferred because of the absence of toxic dyes as well as the ability to reveal colorful toxins which may be excreted in your sweat. On the Testimonials page of our website, we display pads from some of our clients and patients who produced various interesting colors in their sweat!

Ben B. had yellow-green material on his pads during the first few days of his protocol. They may have been chemicals used to clean a cement truck tumbler.

The most fascinating example was from a First Responder of 9/11 who was treated during the *New York Rescue Workers Detoxification Project*. His towels were stained purple. It was so unusual that swatches were sent out for chemical testing. The results came back as toxic manganese. Manganese, found in the dust around Ground Zero, is used in the manufacturing of steel to increase hardness, stiffness, and strength.

Sleep

It is extremely important to get enough sleep to allow time for your body to recover. Sleep will come easier after the first few days. Due to the increased volume of toxicants mobilized in your body and the change to your daily routine, Detoxination may cause side effects in the beginning, such as insomnia, headache, fatigue, nausea, and diarrhea or constipation. Push yourself through the discomfort! Drinking plenty of fluids and replenishing electrolytes will minimize these effects.

Blood Pressure

We monitor blood pressure daily. High heat can have unpredictable effects on blood pressure. People with hypertension should consult with their physician before using a sauna.

Training Heart Rate

Before you begin your Detoxination Program, you should calculate your Training Heart Rate range for optimal exercise output. When you keep your heart rate within this range during exercise, your body will be in the fat-burning zone. Fat burn assists the body with the lipolysis-release of toxins from fat cells.

Training Heart Rate Calculation

This method of monitoring exercise intensity calculates the Training Heart Rate (THR) as a percentage of an age-based theoretical Maximum Heart Rate (MHR). The formula to calculate THR is:

220 – your age = _____ (MHR)

60% of MHR would be the low end of your THR

85% of MHR would be the high end of your THR

Example: 50 years old

220

-50   (Age)

170   (MHR)

x .6   (60% intensity)

102   (low end of THR)

220

-50   (Age)

170   (MHR)

x .85   (85% intensity)

145   (high end of THR)

So, the THR for a 50-year-old would be between 102 and 145 beats per minute. Your fitness level would dictate where in this range you want your heart rate to fall. Previously sedentary individuals would want an intensity level that initially keeps them at the low end of the range, while an active, fit individual would work out higher in the range.

Obviously, the MHR calculated this way is theoretical and only an estimate. Many factors could influence whether an individual's true MHR is higher or lower than that. For instance, recent research has shown that age and gender differences can result in MHR variability of as much as 10 – 12 beats per minute. Beta blockers slow your heart rate, which can prevent the increase in heart rate that typically occurs with exercise.

Daily Routine (FIR Sauna Summary)

- Consume your niacin dose two hours before your session
- Fill out Daily Report Form*
- Record amount of sleep* (See Session Notes)
- Take blood pressure* (See page 176)
- Weigh-in and record* (we monitor how much fluid is sweated out to know how much to replenish)
- Take your initial temperature* (if feverish, skip the day)
- Take lecithin gel cap (per product instruction)
- Drink 4 tablespoons of polyunsaturated, cold pressed oils with a tablespoon of cranberry juice
- Aerobic exercise 20-30 minutes* (jogging, treadmill, exercycle, rebounder, etc.)
- Drink a teaspoon of activated charcoal mixed with 12 ounces water
- Sauna* for 45 minutes for the first of two cycles.
- Take temperature upon exiting sauna and record*
- Replenish electrolytes
- Cool down 15 minutes (cold shower ideal to remove surface toxicants excreted in sweat); optionally incorporate 10 minutes of exercise (try resistance band repetitions)
- Sauna* for 30 minutes and consume 12-16 oz. of Cal-Mag
- Record body temperature immediately upon exiting sauna*
- Replenish electrolytes
- Weigh out and record* (Did you drink enough water?)
- Wash off excreted toxins to avoid reabsorption
- Drink 1 tbsp. Bentonite or micronized zeolite clay with a cup of water

* Recording of vitals and log sheets required if participating in our *Get Detoxinated!* Program. Sample forms available in the Appendix.

Daily Routine (Suggested Dry Sauna Summary)

- Consume your niacin dose two hours before your session
- Fill out Daily Report Form*
- Record amount of sleep* (See Session Notes)
- Take blood pressure* (See page 176)
- Weigh-in and record* (we monitor how much fluid is sweated out to know how much to replenish)
- Take your initial temperature* (if feverish, skip the day)
- Take lecithin gel cap (per product instruction)
- Drink 4 tablespoons of polyunsaturated, cold pressed oils with a tablespoon of cranberry juice
- Aerobic exercise 20-30 minutes* (jogging, treadmill, exercycle, rebounder, etc.)
- Drink a teaspoon of activated charcoal mixed with 12 ounces water
- Sauna* for 15-20 minutes for the first of six sauna cycles.
- Cool down for 5 minutes
- Sauna* for 15-20 minutes for the second of six sauna cycles.
- Take temperature upon exiting sauna and record*
- Replenish electrolytes
- Cool down 15 minutes (cold shower ideal to remove surface toxicants excreted in sweat)
- Sauna* for 15-20 minutes and consume 12-16 oz. of Cal-Mag on the third of six sauna cycles
- Cool down for 5 minutes
- Sauna* for 15-20 minutes for the fourth of six sauna cycles.
- Record body temperature immediately upon exiting sauna*
- Replenish electrolytes
- Cool down 15 minutes (cold shower ideal to remove surface toxicants excreted in sweat); optionally incorporate 10 minutes of exercise (try resistance band repetitions)

- Sauna* for 15-20 minutes for the fifth of six sauna cycles.
- Cool down for 5 minutes
- Sauna* for 15-20 minutes for the sixth of six sauna cycles.
- Take temperature upon exiting sauna and record*
- Replenish electrolytes
- Weigh out and record* (Did you drink enough water?)
- Wash off excreted toxins to avoid reabsorption
- Drink 1 tbsp. Bentonite or micronized zeolite clay with a cup of water

* Recording of vitals and log sheets required if participating in our *Get Detoxinated!* Program. Sample forms available in the Appendix.

Sample Scenarios

These are fictional scenarios to inspire ideas on how Detoxination can fit into your daily routine:

Diane's Story

Diane is a realtor who has a far infrared sauna in her spare bedroom next to a treadmill and rebounder. She sets her alarm for 5 a.m. so she can take the 200 mg niacin dose stirred into a small glass of water that she had just prepared. Diane observes that it will probably take another 4 days before she hits her Target Niacin Dose of 621 milligrams that she calculated based on her weight of 137 pounds. That is, of course, assuming that she only increases her niacin dose by 100 mg per day. Diane then kisses her husband good night. But before she can fall asleep, she wonders what Day 2 of her protocol will be like. She replays her morning in her mind and drifts off to sleep with a great sense of accomplishment for starting on her Detoxination protocol.

At 5 a.m. she drinks her morning niacin dose that is waiting for her on the bedside table, and then she makes herself breakfast. By 5:30 a.m. the powdered niacin has fully bloomed into a bright red flush in her face, chest, and shoulders—from what she can see in the bathroom mirror. Although it was itchy at first, this diminished by 6:15 a.m. when she went to wake up her daughter for school. Her daughter snickered at Mommy's red face, but she has already become used to Mommy's "lobster face," (as she calls it!).

Diane then takes her lecithin gel cap and prepares her vitamins, minerals, and electrolytes for the day's session while her daughter gets ready for school. At 6:45 a.m. she sets the two Dixie cups of electrolytes next the sauna and puts a clean, absorbent pad on the wooden bench. Her daughter gives Diane a hug before running out the front door to catch her school bus. Diane's husband, a chef in an upscale restaurant, then kisses her goodbye on his way out of the house and into his busy work day.

Now home alone at 7 a.m., Diane changes into her workout clothes, turns on the sauna, and then begins walking on their treadmill. Being 31 years old, Diane calculated her Training Heart Rate range to be between 113 and 161 beats per minute, so she periodically checks her heart rate with the built-in monitor on the treadmill.

Not a very athletic person, Diane only pushes herself to 20 minutes of exercise on this second day of her Detoxination program. She then goes into the kitchen and mixes a tablespoon of activated charcoal in a cup of water before quickly drinking it down.

At 7:25 a.m. Diane puts on her robe after undressing, and then she fills her stainless steel drinking canister with 16 oz. of filtered water. She also fills the electric tea kettle with water and then turns it on. Making her way back to the spare bedroom, she steps into the bathroom to weigh herself on the scale next to the tub. Pleased with her maintained weight, she puts the infrared thermometer into her ear canal while pressing the start button. A few seconds later, her temperature boldly appears on the LCD display.

After recording her blood pressure, Diane grabs a hand towel, steps into the sauna, and then adjusts the timer to 45 minutes. Before she makes herself comfortable, Diane places her water canister on the floor by the cooler air near the door, and grabs her tablet.

Once seated, Diane begins checking her email and responding to her clients. Being a workaholic, she is grateful for the far infrared sauna because of her ability to work while doing the protocol. Off in the kitchen she can hear the tea kettle whistling, and a few seconds later she hears the "click" from the auto-shutoff switch. She knows the water will stay plenty warm in that insulated teapot for the remaining 30 minutes before she can attempt her second batch of Cal-Mag.

After taking care of business, Diane brings up YouTube to watch a few videos. Her body is really sweating now, so she begins drawing the hand towel up her legs, then her arms, and up her torso ensuring that her toweling is directed towards her heart. She remembered reading about that in the book, and how it helps to mobilize the lymph system.

At the 45 minute mark, her sauna announces with an audible series of beeps that her first sauna cycle has completed. After restarting the sauna for her next cycle, Diane towels off the remaining sweat and then reaches for the Dixie cup of electrolytes prepared with four cell salt pills, one sodium chloride salt pill, and a potassium capsule. Diane drinks all those down and heads back to the kitchen to prepare the Cal-Mag beverage. On the way back to the kitchen, Diane once again stops in the bathroom to take her temperature. The thermometer shows she raised her core body temperature by two degrees, and it certainly feels like it!

Back in the kitchen, Diane follows the Cal-Mag instructions more closely today. Not one to bake—or even cook for that matter—very often, her first attempt, yesterday, produced an unbearably bad batch! She had mixed up the teaspoon and tablespoon measurements, so her first concoction contained more than twice the magnesium carbonate and too little calcium gluconate. She decided to dump it down the drain and forego her daily Cal-Mag on that first day.

Once correctly mixed and chilled, Diane fills her stainless steel drinking canister and adds a couple of ounces of 100% organic cranberry juice. Next Diane opens the bottle of organic hemp oil and organic flax seed oil to mix her daily cup of cold pressed, polyunsaturated oils. With a tablespoon in hand, she pours two tablespoons each of the oils into a cup, and then splashes a tablespoon of the cranberry juice on top. Tossing the oils down her throat like a shot of tequila, she has found, bypasses the taste buds!

Diane notices she has another 5 minutes before her 15-minute cooldown period ends, so she decides to do a little rebounding to get the blood pumping a bit more. Diane understands that the exercise helps to push the mobilized toxins out towards the dermis layers of skin to aid with their release from her body with her sweat.

With her cool-off break completed, she re-enters the sauna at 8:30 a.m. and sets the timer for 30 minutes. This time Diane brought in a pen and a clipboard with the Detoxination Daily Report and Daily Log forms attached. Before she begins sweating too much to write, she documents her starting weight, temperature before beginning this session, her temperature from the first sauna cycle, her food intake from all her meals since the prior session, any manifestations from the niacin. And, she answers all the other questions on these two forms as completely as possible for the **Get Detoxinated!** Program.

Upon completion of the second sauna cycle, Diane consumes her second Dixie cup full of electrolytes and then records her final temperature. She then weighs out on the bathroom scale before taking a shower to wash off the excreted toxins from her sweaty skin.

Diane then dresses and mixes up a micronized zeolite clay beverage to help her natural detoxification pathways to capture mobilized toxins that permeated back into her GI tract and her bloodstream. Afterwards, Diane prepares her next niacin dose and consumes the vitamins and minerals before heading off to her realty office.

On the third day of the protocol, Diane begins to experience headaches, a little nausea at times, and she didn't sleep well last night. She rereads the section on niacin in the book and realizes that the niacin has mobilized a lot of toxins, and these symptoms confirm how well the Detoxination protocol is actually working!

Since her body is reacting so strongly, Diane decides to stay at the same niacin dose for another day, and pushes on through the protocol. She also plans to consume a cup of activated charcoal at bedtime to help rid her system of the higher volume of toxins that have been coming out of her fat cells. Hopefully, this will help her sleep better.

By the fifth day, Diane is feeling a little better. Her body is still feeling the effects of the toxins, but these symptoms are more tolerable. Diane decides to increase her niacin dose again, but this time her niacin flush reveals white strap marks on her shoulders and upper chest that match a bathing suit she had worn eight years ago! That was when she got sunburned really badly because she fell asleep on her beach towel at West Shore Lake Tahoe!

Fortunately, the niacin-manifested sunburn didn't hurt like the first time, and the strap marks faded away forever along with her flush after 45 minutes. Once the novelty of this bizarre episode wore off, Diane realized that she needed to document her manifestation on her Detoxination Daily Report.

Now well into her second week, Diane is beginning to feel better about her daily routine and overall sense of wellbeing. It took her 11 days to reach her Target Niacin Dose. Now that she attained that goal, her plan is to continue increasing her niacin by 100 mg until day 14.

She is finally getting eight hours of sleep, and she can remember her dreams! The other obvious change is how well food tastes now. Even the smells of the individual ingredients are stronger. Diane is also noticing colors are different—they're more vivid!

Diane learned early on to drink at least 40 ounces of water to stay properly hydrated during the protocol, so she no longer feels lightheaded, fatigued, or dizzy while in the sauna. Sometimes she feels she needs more electrolytes, so she will double up after her second sauna cycle on those days. She will also add another potassium capsule when she feels like her body needs it.

Diane completes her protocol in 16 days. She decides to go a couple more days to taper down from the 1,100 mg niacin she achieved at the end. Of course, she still follows the vitamins and minerals schedule based on her niacin dose even while tapering down.

A month after completing her protocol, Diane's friends are amazed at how well she looks and how she seems more alert and focused. She tells her friends that she feels wonderful and *young* again!

Jack's Scenario

Jack is a plumber who decides to use the sauna at the gym for his Detoxination protocol. He plans to go after work each day for the three hours it'll take to do the protocol in their dry sauna. As much as he'd like to own a sauna, he just can't afford it right now. Besides, his studio apartment wouldn't accommodate even a 1-person sauna anyway.

By going to the gym, Jack will have to prepare everything in advance, such as the Cal-Mag, oils, electrolytes, and niacin. He will carry them in re-usable containers, along with his workout attire, in his gym bag. Jack was smart to purchase a Berkey® Sports Bottle for filtering water from the faucet so he doesn't have to carry water with him every day. He likes having the built-in filter that purifies his drinking water as he drinks from the special straw.

Since Jack gets off work at 5 p.m., he takes his niacin dose at 3:30 p.m.—timing the rebound lipolysis with his arrival at the gym. His co-workers chided him at first for the niacin flush, but he found that his clients were quite supportive when he explained why he was red on his amply exposed skin!

Beginning his protocol at 5:45—after checking in at the gym and getting changed—Jack takes a lecithin gel cap and drinks his cold pressed, polyunsaturated oils. He then begins 30 minutes of low-impact aerobic exercises starting on the exercycle. After 10 minutes, he switches to the treadmill for another 10 minutes before completing the half-hour workout on the elliptical machine.

Fortunately, the sauna is usually occupied so he doesn't have to pre-heat it. Jack is silently thankful that he doesn't have to maintain the sauna, either, but the thought is soon replaced by sudden apprehension. He makes a mental note to inquire into the gym's policies and procedures for cleaning—and sterilizing—their saunas!

Since Jack has chosen not to participate in the **Get Detoxinated!** Program, he doesn't need to record as much information. He will, however, jot down his niacin dosages, his intake of vitamins and minerals, and record any manifestations during the protocol. Each day he will weigh himself in and weigh himself out to ensure that he is staying appropriately hydrated, as well.

Before entering the sauna, Jack drinks the activated charcoal mixed with water from a little glass jar, then grabs his hand towel that he brought from home. He doesn't like the ones provided by the gym because they smell of industrial-strength laundry detergent. Jack figures if he's in for a penny, he's going in for a pound. He doesn't want to add to his toxic body burden with their cleaning chemicals, if he can help it.

Jack also brings into the sauna his pill bottles containing the electrolytes as well as his Berkey® Sports Bottle he just filled with tap water. He steps into the sauna at the very moment another occupant dowses the heated stones with water. Suddenly an oppressively hot cloud of steam wafts over him as he struggles to find a seat on the lower bench.

The steam feels good, though, and Jack settles in for a 15-minute sauna bath—the first of six 15-minute cycles he plans to do. Jack is aware that dry, or convection, saunas are not as efficient in generating sebaceous sweat as far infrared saunas; therefore, he figures he will need to do at least 90 minutes, overall, in these saunas. Jack has set up a workable sauna schedule to achieve the desired results during his Detoxination Program:

Activity	Minutes	Additional Actions
Sauna Cycle 1	15	Drink activate charcoal with water
Cool Down	5	Towel off toxins
Sauna Cycle 2	15	Stay Hydrated
Shower/Cool off	15	Take electrolytes
Sauna Cycle 3	15	Drink Cal-Mag during sauna
Cool Down	5	Towel off toxins
Sauna Cycle 4	15	Stay Hydrated
Shower/Treadmill	15	Take electrolytes
Sauna Cycle 5	15	Stay Hydrated
Cool Down	5	Towel off toxins
Sauna Cycle 6	15	Stay Hydrated
Shower/Dress		Take electrolytes

With this schedule, Jack will shower off the toxins eliminated with his sweat after each 30 minutes of sauna time. In addition, he will take his stainless steel canister of Cal-Mag into the sauna to drink during the third sauna cycle. Jack will also consume his electrolytes after each 30 minutes of sauna time, so he prepared three pill bottles each containing four cell salts, one sodium chloride pill, and one potassium pill.

Jack has also elected to increase his circulation with a brief, 10-minute walk on a treadmill before beginning his fifth sauna cycle. All-in-all, this is a very well-thought-out plan. He will take his vitamins and minerals once he gets home.

During his sauna cycles, Jack sits on a white gym towel. With his gym shorts on in the sauna, he's less concerned with the laundry soap on their towels. In fact, he's been noticing that his towels are stained each day with a yellow-green material that smells like old, coconut suntan oil he used two summers ago!

But after 5 days on this schedule, the stains are gone—along with the smell of coconut oil. Jack has been paying very close attention to how his body reacts to these daily sessions. He recalled the book discussing strange manifestations caused by niacin, but he wasn't prepared for the next big one that happened the very next day!

Well into the third sauna cycle on his sixth day, Jack suddenly notices that his left ankle is swollen. Although not painful, the swelling appeared in the exact location of an injury he had sustained during his final football game of the high school season! The sprain was so bad that he never took to the field again.

On this day, he decides to not walk on the treadmill before his fourth sauna cycle, but he needn't worry—the swelling is gone by then.

Jack completed his Detoxination Program in 21 days, and even though he experienced some diarrhea in the beginning and a few headaches along the way, his "End Phenomenon" was very obvious.

Four months later and he's feeling great and sleeping even better. He is pleased that his weight is so much easier to maintain, as well!

Frequently Asked Questions – FAQs
Q. I don't sweat. Can I do the protocol?

Sweat glands aid your body in cooling down and regulating your temperature. They also put salt back into your bloodstream and relieve muscles of excess heat. Decreased sweating, or hypohidrosis, can have some serious repercussions such as heat stroke or even death in severe cases.

If you have been diagnosed with a medical condition that leads to hypohidrosis, consult with your practitioner before initiating the protocol.

We have seen many cases where pores and hair follicles are simply clogged; and after several days on the protocol the individual begins to sweat profusely. Try sauna with increasing durations over a few days to see if your body can produce sweat. Take 50-100 mg of niacin on one of those days to see if the vasodilation aids in opening your pores and follicles.

Do not do the protocol if you fail to produce sweat after three days.

Q. I have bad knees. Do I have to exercise?

The exercise component is designed to get blood to circulate the mobilized toxins into the dermis layers of the skin. From there the sauna portion of the protocol can eliminate the toxins via sweat.

If you cannot tolerate exercise due to bad knees or other condition, then other options are available.

One suggestion is to use a rebounder with a handle (mini-trampoline). Another is to purchase the BodyGym or other resistance band product to move your other muscles.

If you can tolerate a bicycle or exercycle, then go with this preferred option.

Interestingly, many people with knee pain find sauna therapy actually relieves the pain after a few sessions.

Q. I have breast implants. Can I do the protocol?

You may want to consult with your practitioner before using a sauna or doing the protocol, but we have no problems related to implants.

Breast implants, whether saline- or gel-filled, will heat up during sauna, less so in a far infrared or full spectrum infrared sauna than a convection sauna. Your body will cool down much faster than the breast implants after sauna, but they will never get hot enough to become damaged. It would take temperatures of 200°C (392°F) in order to melt breast implants, so you would likely be dead before the breast implant became a problem!

Q. I have a MTHFR mutation. Can I do the protocol?

Yes. The gene mutation may cause methylation issues affecting your detoxification pathways, so this protocol is especially warranted. Reducing your toxic exposures and your body burden through sweat decreases the load placed on the liver.

With MTHRF, you should pay closer attention to these signs:

- Dizziness
- Light-headedness
- Feeling faint
- Intense fatigue
- Excessively hot
- Very fast heart rate

At the first sign of intolerable levels of any of these symptoms, get out of the sauna and stop the protocol for that day. Don't push yourself, but be aware that these symptoms may be signs that the protocol is working to mobilize toxins, and are to be expected.

For more advice on sauna with MTHFR, Dr. Ben Lynch provides an excellent article on the topic at http://mthfr.net/benefits-of-sauna/2015/01/13/.

Q. How often should I be doing the protocol?

After completing the full protocol, we recommend a maintenance protocol every few years. In order to build on the gains from this protocol, we recommend spending 30 minutes in a sauna every other day. If you don't have a sauna, but would like to own one, we can help you select the most appropriate one for your needs.

I personally do a 5-day version of the protocol every six months in order to stay healthy, alert, focused, and feeling great! It is a great way to recover from a less-than-"purefect" lifestyle, too!

Q. My blood tests are higher after the protocol, why?

Believe it or not, that is a great sign that the protocol is working! If you recall from Chapter 1, my father's research demonstrated that the fat cells are 200-500 times more toxic than blood serum tests reveal. Therefore, after you complete the protocol and have your blood tested, the levels indicate that some xenobiotics, which have been pulled from the fat, are still circulating in the blood.

If your blood serum levels of xenobiotics are still high, then you should consider continuing the protocol or, at minimum, continue with binders like Bentonite clay, zeolite clay, or activated charcoal.

Q. What kind of sauna should I use/buy?

Saunas come in a variety of formats, including traditional convection, far infrared (FIR), full spectrum infrared, and sauna cabinets. Although most any sauna will suffice for the protocol, some are definitely more desirable than others.

We do not recommend steam rooms for several reasons. First, they are not sanitary. Bacteria and fungi—which prefer damp, warm environments—are easily transmitted to you on the steam. Also, steam readily transports toxins from others to you. Finally, steam saturates the air so much, that sweat doesn't easily evaporate off the body. Like convection saunas, steam is less efficient than infrared sauna for detoxification, and you spend more time in those unsanitary conditions. Never the less, if steam is the best you've got to work with, the upside outweighs the downsides!

I had to decide which sauna manufacturer delivered the best value and could stand up to the demands of our Detoxination Protocol. As I delved further into my research, heater types, wood choices, ease of use, seating options, warranty, and aesthetics all became important considerations.

In addition, issues of EMFs (Electro Magnetic Frequencies) and off-gassing of Volatile Organic Compounds (VOCs) inherent in low quality units had to be addressed. Can't add more toxins or toxic conditions to our clients or patients!

After careful review, we confidently selected the Jacuzzi® Sauna Sanctuary line for our centers. These are their full spectrum units, that provide near, mid, and far infrared wavelengths to provide greater therapeutic benefits.

Convection saunas have historically been the sauna used the most by practitioners of the Hubbard Method, and they are quite capable of the task. However, we encountered some issues when we were still working with traditional dry saunas:

- More time to reach desired temperature
- More time to heat the body (which added time to the protocol)
- Shorter tolerable sauna sessions (10-15 minutes at 180°F)
- 4.3 times less toxin elimination than with full spectrum infrared
- Less energy efficient, therefore more expensive to use

Once we made the switch to Far Infrared sauna, we found significant decreases in program times and increases in xenobiotic reductions. The utility costs were also decreased and the overall experience was greatly enhanced.

To learn more about the history of saunas, different heating methods (including FIR), and the best materials for different types of heat therapy, we recommend the book by Dr. Nenah Sylver, *The Holistic Handbook of Sauna Therapy*. If you wish to purchase this book or need a sauna to complete the protocol, please visit our website store at https://www.GetDetoxinated.com/shop/.

Q. What temperature do you recommend?

Temperature is a matter of tolerance. You should eventually be able to sauna for 45 minutes in the first of two cycles; therefore work your way up to that duration as quickly as possible. Convection saunas tend to average 180°F, and most individuals can only tolerate that level of oppressive heat for 10-20 minutes at a time.

The goal is to sweat... and to sweat a lot! We find that most people will sweat around 130-140°F, and if you're using an infrared sauna, your ability to stay longer in the heat is far better.

Q. Since EMF is a problem, how can I get it tested?

First of all, not all electromagnetic fields (or frequencies) are bad. For instance, far infrared saunas use a good form of EMF to produce molecular vibrations within your cells to create heat.

Electromagnetic frequencies can be used to heal the body from everything from pathogens to cancers. Dr. Royal Rife, inventor of the Rife Frequency Machine, identified the resonant frequency (the frequency that pathogens vibrate) to cause tiny organisms to oscillate to a point that they would either be shut down or destroyed.

In her book, *The Rife Handbook of Frequency Therapy and Holistic Health*, Nenah Sylver PhD provides an excellent history and instructions for the use of Rife Frequency devices—and it is an invaluable reference manual for holistic therapies *and living* in general!

But there are harmful types EMF, called *electrosmog,* that we encounter daily from too many sources. Thousands of studies link low-level electromagnetic frequency radiation exposures to a long list of adverse biological effects, including:

- Oxidative damage
- Disruption of cell metabolism
- Increased blood brain barrier permeability
- Melatonin reduction

The newest offending EMF is called 5G. This new wireless technology requires many more towers producing much more EMF radiation.

Many sauna manufacturers use inferior, toxic materials that off-gas volatile organic compounds to construct their units, and their heaters are usually of similar, poor quality. As such the electrosmog radiation from these units should be avoided.

The preferred method for testing EMF as well as microwave radiation is the Trifield TF2 meter at around $168. This meter will detect harmful radiation from electromagnetic fields as well as cellphones, wifi routers, and other wireless devices.

For the cost-conscious individual, we recommend the Meterk EMF Meter Electromagnetic Field Radiation Detector for around $33. It will tell you if the target sauna is producing safe or unsafe levels of electromagnetic fields.

Q. Doesn't niacin cause liver damage?

Pure nicotinic acid is the immediate release form of niacin, and is considered the safest form. All other forms of niacin are either incapable of producing the desired rebound lipolysis or are damaging to the liver. This includes niacinamide (aka nicotinamide), inositol hexanicotinate, and the hepatoxic form called sustained-release niacin.

We only recommend the crystalline form of pure nicotinic acid for the protocol. However, the pill-form is acceptable in the first few days. As you titrate up to your Target Niacin Dose of 10 mg/kg, the crystalline form is more practical. Switching from the pill to the powder form can cause immediate nausea, and this is why we start individuals on the powdered form of niacin.

Q. Is there a good or bad time of day to take niacin?

Actually, no, there isn't a preferred time of day to take the niacin as long as it is taken 2 hours before your session. It should be noted, however, that you want to try to be consistent with the times you start each day. Don't worry if you can't be too consistent with your start times, but try your best anyway.

Keep in mind, though, that the vitamins and minerals should be replenished according to the schedules beginning on page127, so do not begin the protocol late at night if you can help it.

Q. I don't always get a niacin flush, is that ok?

Absolutely it is OK! Vasodilation from the niacin flush helps open the capillaries and gets blood circulating into the tissues, but the lack of flushing isn't going to affect rebound lipolysis or your session gains.

Don't sweat it (pardon the pun!) if you aren't having the flush. Just increase your niacin dose for the full benefits.

Q. Niacin gives me the chills. Is this normal?

Chills or shivering can be caused by the dissipation of heat from open capillaries during the niacin flush causing a thermal energy exchange to the surrounding air. The heat is replaced by cooler air just like how an air conditioner evaporator and condenser work.

Q. I use supplements regularly. Why do I need to take more?

Great question! The vitamins and minerals schedule provided earlier are based on the average losses, due to sweat, of these vital nutrients based on the current niacin dose. Therefore, rather than thinking of these as "supplements," think of them as "replenishments."

The schedule of replenishments should bring you back to a safe level of these vitamins and minerals. Do not increase these vitamins and minerals, but you may continue with other supplements and herbs not included in the tables on pages 128 and 129.

Q. When should I take the supplements?

The vitamins and minerals synergistically work together and should be consumed soon after your session. Some vitamins become more bioavailable with food in your stomach. Fat soluble vitamins, including A, D, K, and E, need fatty acids for absorption, so pair foods that are rich in these nutrients with a source of healthy fat, like nuts or oil.

To prevent an imbalance or "secondary deficiencies" of other vitamins, avoid excessive dosing of B vitamins. The Vitamins and Minerals Tables provided on pages 128 and 129 are the recommended dosages for each range of vitamin B3 (niacin) ingested.

Q. How much Cal-Mag should I consume?

Try to consume at least 12-16 oz. during your session. We provide Cal-Mag during the second, 30-minute cycle and it is included in the total hydration figure recorded each day.

Q. Is it OK to do the protocol alone?

Yes. For safety sake, it is best to have someone periodically check in on you while you're in the sauna. It is better to have a partner doing the protocol with you.

Watch for signs of dehydration or depleted electrolytes. These include clammy skin, weakness or extreme tiredness, headaches, nausea, cramps, vomiting, and fainting.

When I am doing the protocol alone in our FIR sauna, I have my cellphone with me. To check up on me, Suzy can text me periodically. If I fail to respond, she can take action to ensure I'm okay.

CHAPTER 4
Sustainable Health

After completing Detoxination you are a relatively clean slate, so let's work to keep your body that way!

And, you deserve our sincerest *congratulations!*

Remember, we're bombarded daily by toxins from all kinds of sources, so I am going to now share with you ways that we minimize our toxin exposures for sustainable health.

This is by no means a complete list; it is just a starting point for you to build upon in your own life.

Cooking and Kitchen
Pots and Pans

The material used to add a non-stick coating to frying pans or skillets is a fluropolymer, like polytetrafluoroetheylene (PTFE) which we know as Teflon. While Teflon is convenient for cleanup, it is highly toxic to the body. When heated during cooking, PTFE becomes a source for perfluorooctanoic acid (PFOA) which has been linked to a wide range of health problems including thyroid disease, infertility in women, organ damage, and developmental and reproductive problems.

Even though the US Environmental Protection Agency (EPA) has declared perfluorinated compounds (PFCs) to be "likely carcinogens" these chemicals are still used in a wide array of household products. A study conducted by the Centers for Disease Control and Prevention (CDC) discovered that roughly 98% of Americans now have traces of PFA's or PFC's in their bodies.

Manufacturers were required to eliminate PFOA from cooking products back in 2015.

Aluminum is no better. Aluminum, a toxic heavy metal, is absorbed into all foods cooked in it and it is released from the cooked food into our bodies. Aluminum has been associated with estrogen-related disorders, including cancers, and Alzheimer's Disease.

Better solutions, not in any particular order, include:

Ceramic - glazed ceramic cookware is durable, heat efficient and environmentally friendly as well, but it can easily chip. Recent concerns have been raised regarding small amounts of lead coming from the porcelain glaze.

Stainless Steel - stainless steel is one of the safest cookware materials in existence, and for many forms of cooking it is an excellent non-stick surface if it's not exposed to high heat. Look for surgical stainless steel.

Cast Iron - cast iron is extremely durable and conducts heat beautifully. It can go from the stovetop to the oven, or be used over any cook source, like outdoor grills and camp fires. Cast iron needs to be properly seasoned, however, and the pans are quite heavy. We do use cast iron at home because we love camping! Cast iron is perfect for portable propane stove cooking. We just wipe out the remaining dregs from the pan and then boil water to clean it.

There are other alternatives, some better than others. Do a little investigative research for yourself to discover what works best for your needs.

Microwaves, Toaster Ovens and Convection Ovens

Microwave cooking became popular in 1946 after Percy Spencer, an inventor, scientist, and radio engineer, discovered that a chocolate bar in his pocket had melted while he was working on radar equipment for Raytheon. In fact, the first microwave ovens were called Radarange for this very reason.

The problems with cooking in a microwave oven include the stripping away of foods' original nutrients, and the adding of toxins to food if it was cooked in plastic containers or wrap. When breast milk is heated in a microwave, the health benefits of vitamin B-12 are instantly negated. Microwave heating of breast milk also destroys the powerful bacteria-fighting agents that can lead to E. coli growth.

Better alternatives include toaster ovens and convection ovens.

Storage of Leftovers and Other Foods

Tupperware and similar food storage containers are typically made with BPA and/or phthalate containing plastics, which should be replaced by much safer glass or stainless steel containers.

Certainly you should stop microwaving foods altogether, but if you must reheat stored food in a microwave, don't do it in plastic containers. Good Pyrex glassware, which is made with non-toxic tempered soda-lime glass, can usually withstand extreme thermal changes from refrigerator to the microwave oven.

Water Filtration

There are many water filtration products on the market, and it can be tough to decide which system is the best fit for your needs. While choosing the best purifier to reduce or remove viruses, bacteria, cysts, sand, silt, sediment, chemicals, organic compounds, pesticides, heavy metals, fluoride, chlorine and chloramines, you must also determine what format will be most cost-effective in the long run.

There are pitchers, gravity fed charcoal or ceramic filters, under sink filters and whole house filters. Additionally, you have multi-stage filter systems, distillation units, reverse osmosis filters, alkalinizers, and ultraviolet water purifiers. And don't forget the shower filter to remove chlorine gas!

For the purpose of hydration while on the Detoxination protocol, we use a gravity-fed charcoal filter in our centers, as well as at home. They are very economical and produce great tasting, filtered water.

Distillation systems produce the purest water; however, all the beneficial minerals are removed. They also do not reduce volatile organic compounds or endocrine disrupting chemicals, such as fluoride, very well. We recommend adding 1-2 tbsp. of apple cider vinegar to a gallon of distilled water for many health benefits.

Whole house water filters are a great investment, especially if you can get the filters to reduce or remove fluoride. Reverse osmosis has long been established as a great water filtration system, but it does require a lot of maintenance. Even chlorine can damage an RO system, so a pre-filter is usually installed. Also, RO requires annual filter changes, periodic backwashes to clean the filter, and sterilization. Some RO systems are very inefficient and can discharge 84% of the water into the sewer! For every 3 gallons of water processed, only 1 gallon is usable filtered water. Look for "zero-discharge" systems when purchasing an RO filter.

With all the available products on the market, researching the pros and cons of each type is time well spent. For a thorough exploration of water and filtering methods, see chapter three in *The Rife Handbook of Frequency Therapy and Holistic Health* by Nenah Sylver PhD.

Our online store has links to Dr. Sylver's books and our preferred brands of water filter systems and accessories at:

https://www.GetDetoxinated.com/shop/.

Ice Maker

While we're on the topic of water, consider purchasing a stand-alone ice maker and fill it with your filtered water. Built-in freezer ice makers are convenient, but the filters are often neglected and they aren't as effective in reducing the contaminants that make us sick.

Vegetable Garden and Fruit Trees

Many years ago we planted fruit trees along our fence and set up raised vegetable garden beds. It is very rewarding to grow your own organic produce and teach your kids how to care for a garden. We also have friends who have done the same, so we share in our bounties.

If you can carve out even a small area to plant vegetables, you will save money and find the fruits and vegetables actually taste better!

But be sure to avoid using any toxic herbicides or pesticides in your garden. Manually weed your garden beds, and to kill unwanted aphids try releasing ladybugs! Baby ladybugs devour about 400 aphids, and in their lifetime may consume over 5,000 of these plant-consuming pests.

When it comes to soil, especially box-store bags of soil, you should add your own natural fertilizers such as worm castings, animal manure, and remnants of plant matter. Composting is a great way to recycle your organic kitchen scraps, and helps rebuild nutrients in the soil.

Smoothies

We drink a lot of fruit and veggie smoothies in our household. Suzy purchases organic produce items when we haven't grown them ourselves, and then cuts them up into small chunks that she then freezes for later use.

I always find it amazing how well things taste blended together without following recipes! Plus, the frozen produce replaces the need for ice.

Even my kids like to make their own smoothie before school!

Grooming
Salt Stick Deodorant

Consider replacing your deodorant with a Thai Crystal Deodorant Stone. These mineral salt sticks contain no paraben, oils, fragrances, emulsifiers or aluminum chlorhydrate, and are hypoallergenic.

I have been using these Thai Crystal stones for years and love how they kill the odor-causing bacteria.

Homemade Toothpaste and Tom's of Maine

For your teeth, why not make your own, fluoride-free and non-toxic toothpaste? Here's the recipe we use:

Coconut Oil Toothpaste

One tsp baking soda sifted into a small bowl
One tbsp. coconut oil (creamed)
Mix together in a small, lidded jar
You can also add:
Peppermint oil
Activated charcoal – 3 caps
Turmeric – 3 caps
¼ tsp peroxide

If you prefer to use an off-the-shelf product, we recommend Tom's Of Maine brand of natural toothpaste. Make sure to check the label to ensure that you are purchasing fluoride-free versions.

Body Wash, Shampoo, and Conditioner

The Environmental Working Group maintains the Skin Deep Database which ranks skin care products based on their toxicity. This is a great resource; however, they have come under fire recently for being alarmist to garner media attention.

Because of loopholes in federal law, skin care and cosmetic brands are able to make claims like "natural," "non-toxic," and "organic" without regulations. Therefore, these terms have become meaningless.

Avoid products that contain parabens, sodium lauryl sulfate, and propylene glycol. If a product claims to be organic, look for the certified USDA Organic seal.

There are manufacturers who have stepped up to produce chemical-free, organic body products, and you can find our favorite brands in our online store.

Shaving Cream

Shaving cream manufacturers are notorious for using noxious chemicals to dispense their products. They also use chemicals to prepare the skin and hair for the razor. Here's what we suggest you look for in non-toxic shaving cream:

- Fragrance Free on the label
- Few ingredients
- Natural oils, like coconut, jojoba, or olive oil

Aloe is always a plus Here's what *not* to find in shaving cream:

- *Sulfates* which create the lather
- *Propylene Glycol* commonly used as a moisturizer, but is also added to brake fluid and antifreeze!
- *Triethanolamine* (TES) is an emulsifier which prevents oil and water from separating, but is linked to cancer and is a hormone disrupting toxin.
- *Fragrance* should always be avoided as they tend to be artificial chemicals blended together.
- *Canned* shaving products use aerosols to dispense the product, and the foam that's created is caused by chemicals called surfactants. Surfactants interfere with the natural process of hydration.

Recommended products, in price order (high to low), are manufactured by:

- Henry Cavendish
- Pacific Shaving Company
- Dr. Bonners
- Burt's Bees

Chlorine Filter for Shower

Chlorine may be effective at killing water-borne pathogens, but it can upset the delicate balance of the skin microbiome and dry out the largest organ of your body.

Skin absorbs 60 percent of what it comes in contact with, and while under hot water, the pores are wide open to absorbing chlorine in the shower. Chlorine gas can be produced during a hot shower, so you should consider installing a chlorine shower filter.

Laundry and Cleaning

Clean out your cleaning products and use natural ingredients to make your own cleaning and laundry detergent from these recipes:

Household Cleaner

At our Centers and around the house we use a spray bottle with

- ¼ cup of white 5% vinegar
- 1½ cups of distilled water
- 25 drops of lemon essential oil

Simply shake to combine, spray onto surface to be cleaned, and wipe clean.

Window Cleaner

In a spray bottle, add

- ½ cup white 5% vinegar
- ½ cup rubbing alcohol
- 1 tbsp. cornstarch
- 10 drops of lemon essential oil

Shake to combine, spray on windows, mirrors, or glass and then wipe clean with a lint-free cloth.

Laundry

We quit using detergents and bleach to wash clothes several years ago. Instead we have been happily using Laundry Balls as a great, non-toxic substitute. The brand we use is Crystal Wash, and they work by creating higher alkaline water by the agitation while moving around your dirty clothes. This creates a natural hydrogen peroxide-type effect which disinfects you clothes. The Bio Ceramic balls contained in the shells collect the odors, dirt and waste from your laundry. They get recharged when they are put in the sunlight for an afternoon every 30 days or so. Two of these Laundry Balls come in a package and are apparently good for 1,000 loads.

Dryer balls

There are even dryer balls made of wool that work really well to collect lint, reduce wrinkles, and are anti-static. They are very inexpensive and do a wonderful job.

Normal dryer sheets are loaded with toxic chemicals. Most people don't think twice about this anti-static cling and fresh-smelling household product, but the fact is they are probably the worst thing you can do to your clothes that you then put on your body! In addition to harmful fragrances, here seven toxic chemicals and their dangers for your consideration:[109]

---

[109] "7 Toxic Reasons to Ditch Dryer Sheets | Make Your Clothes Healthier." *Healthy Living How To*(blog). August 10, 2017. https://healthylivinghowto.com/healthy-body-7-toxic-reasons-to-ditch-dryer-sheets/.

1. Alpha-Terpineol causes central nervous system disorders. Can also cause loss of muscular coordination, central nervous system depression, and headache.

2. Benzyl Alcohol causes central nervous system disorders, headaches, nausea, vomiting, dizziness, central nervous system depression, and, in severe cases, death.

3. Camphor is on the US EPA's Hazardous Waste list. This central nervous system stimulant causes dizziness, confusion, nausea, twitching muscles, and convulsions.

4. Chloroform is on the EPA's Hazardous Waste list. Neurotoxic and carcinogenic.

5. Ethyl Acetate is on the EPA's Hazardous Waste list. Narcotic. May cause headaches and narcosis (stupor).

6. Linalool causes central nervous system disorders. Narcotic. In studies of animals, it caused ataxic gait (loss of muscular coordination), reduced spontaneous motor activity, and depression.

7. Pentane causes headaches, nausea, vomiting, dizziness, drowsiness, and loss of consciousness. Repeated inhalation of vapors causes central nervous system depression.

Leisure

Sauna

As we discussed in Chapter 2, saunas are ideal for safely and effectively reducing toxins from your body, but they offer many other health benefits as well.

Heat is great for easing pain and reducing sore muscles, improving joint movement, and easing arthritis pain. Sauna heat reduces stress levels and promotes relaxation. Some parents of autistic children put their kids in a sauna before bedtime to help them fall asleep.

The reduction of stress from sauna may be linked to lower risk of cardiovascular events. People with asthma may find relief from sauna as it helps open airways and loosen phlegm. Loosening phlegm was very apparent with the 9/11 First Responders: they brought up much black mucous from their lungs during treatment.

German sauna medical research shows that saunas were able to significantly reduce the incidences of colds and influenza among participants. As the body is exposed to the heat of a sauna and steam (from water applied to heated rocks), it produces white blood cells more rapidly, which in turn help to fight illnesses and kill viruses. In addition, saunas can relieve the uncomfortable symptoms of sinus congestion from colds or allergies.

Professor Abo from Japan confirmed a 40% improvement in the function of the immune system by raising the body temperature by only 1.8° Fahrenheit.

Sauna heat is one of the oldest strategies for cleansing the skin. It rinses the dead skin and bacteria out of the epidermal layer and sweat ducts.

Lastly, having a sauna just feels good! Even people with type II diabetes mellitus gain improvements with Far Infrared saunas.[110]

If you don't already own one, you should consider purchasing the healthiest appliance you can ever add to your home. After

---

[110] Beever, Richard. "The Effects of Repeated Thermal Therapy on Quality of Life in Patients with Type II Diabetes Mellitus." *The Journal of Alternative and Complementary Medicine* 16, no. 6 (2010), 677-681.
https://www.ncbi.nlm.nih.gov/pubmed/20569036?fbclid=IwAR3YY6AWxe5jD_FrpV AQrUkHds59nmISsdYPqN2KmXLlkeHRShY20UK0z4I.

completing the protocol you can continue to maintain your healthy body with just 30 minutes of sauna every other day!

Television

Limit what you watch on television. It is called "programming" for good reason. Your thoughts, emotions, opinions, and stress levels are easily manipulated through the news, commercials, suspense thrillers, and sports.

You've probably heard people say that stress is toxic. I agree with that statement. We have a built-in system to deal with situations of danger, stress, or when otherwise stimulated called the autonomic nervous system. The two parts that matter to television are the sympathetic and parasympathetic nervous systems.

The sympathetic nervous system is what triggers the fight-or-flight mode, and it can even happen with *perceived* threats, such as the anxiety from television programming. When you are in the sympathetic state, the hypothalamus in your brain sends an alarm that releases a surge of hormones to help you react faster. These include adrenaline and cortisol, which would be used up if the threat were real; however, they build to toxic levels when not used.

According to the American Psychological Association, these toxic levels of stress hormones can be directly linked to chronic conditions such as cardiovascular disease, dysregulated metabolism, and increased agitation or irritability. This harmful condition can also impair our emotional well-being and central nervous system.

When we stay in the fight-or-flight mode for extended periods of time, our physical health is not all that is compromised. Chronic elevated stress also negatively impacts learning, creativity, and overall cognition, which isn't a good combination for our health.

So, do like I did and stop watching television altogether. Enjoy the benefits of the parasympathetic mode which promotes growth and regeneration!

Weed and Pest Control

Use non-toxic, environmentally safe pesticides and herbicides, or make your own.

There are many formulas for natural weed killers, and they do work if you are persistent with applications. The one I make and use the most, where I am not growing anything important, uses this recipe:

In a 1-gallon sprayer mix

- ½ gallon 20% white vinegar (household 5% is too weak!)
- 1 cup of table salt
- 1 tablespoon liquid dish soap
- Fill with water

Once you have these ingredients thoroughly mixed, spray the offending weeds with a healthy coating. The liquid soap acts as a surfactant and also helps the mixture to adhere to the weeds. If the weeds are mature or very tall, it is best to cut them down a bit with a weed whacker.

You will have to reapply this homemade weed killer in another week or so. This does not attack the root system, just the leafy parts. It will sterilize the ground around the weeds for a while, so nothing will grow there.

There is also a pre-mixed product that I have successfully used in the past, called BioSafe; however, it is a very expensive solution!

Pests are best handled by adding live ladybugs and spiders into your garden environment. Neither will eat your plants, and they do a wonderful job of pest control!

These are all the "wellness hacks" I have for the book, but you will find more ideas added regularly to our website at the following link:

https://www.GetDetoxinated.com/book/

Also, to get more great information, solutions, and formulas for homemade, non-toxic substitutions for household products emailed weekly, sign up for our Weekly Wellness Hacks at

https://www.getdetoxinated.com/membership-account/membership-levels/

We would love to add your solutions, so please email them to info@GetDetoxinated.com

Please join our online forum on Facebook at:

https://www.facebook.com/groups/Detox.iNation

You may find answers to questions not addressed in this book, testimonials from others, interesting posts and useful information, and a whole lot more!

We ask that you add your testimonial there, too!

CONCLUSION

We have covered a lot of material in this book, yet it is only the tip of the proverbial iceberg of available information on this subject. It is our sincerest hope that you have a better understanding that:

- At the root of most inflammatory, autoimmune, neurological, and endocrine disorders are bioaccumulated toxins that lead to illness-causing inflammation
- Poor nutrition denies the body of critical materials needed to heal itself properly
- The high cost of illness, disease, and cancer is not only bankrupting us financially, but emotionally, as well.
- This solution is neither known nor taught to conventional medical providers, and
- Detoxination is the only safe and effective path to *sustainable* health!

We encourage you to use this knowledge to improve your own quality of life and health, and then share your experience with others. If you don't already have the most powerful health tool at home, then consider either purchasing a sauna or scheduling to come visit us in Sacramento to ***Get Detoxinated!***

You will find most everything you need for the Detoxination Protocol from our online store at https://www.GetDetoxinated.com/shop/.

For those of you interested in going deeper into the science behind sauna detoxification, be sure to read the 50-page report submitted to the California Medical Board in 1987 starting on page 180 of the Appendix.

Health Really Does Control Wealth!

Your Path To Sustainable Health Starts Here!

APPENDIX

Blood Pressure

The following table of blood pressure reference ranges should be used as a guide if you are monitoring and recording blood pressure while on the protocol.

AGE	FEMALE	MALE
15-18	117/77 mmHg	120/85 mmHg
19-24	120/79 mmHg	120/79 mmHg
25-29	120/80 mmHg	121/80 mmHg
30-35	122/81 mmHg	123/82 mmHg
36-39	123/82 mmHg	124/83 mmHg
40-45	124/83 mmHg	125/83 mmHg
46-49	126/84 mmHg	127/84 mmHg
50-55	129/85 mmHg	128/85 mmHg
56-59	130/86 mmHg	131/87 mmHg
60 and older	134/84 mmHg	135/88 mmHg

High blood pressure, also known as hypertension, is diagnosed when your systolic blood pressure is routinely above 140 or your diastolic pressure is above 90. Because high heat can have unpredictable effects on blood pressure, people with hypertension should consult a medical expert before using a sauna.

Sample Forms

The *Detoxination Daily Log*, on page 178, is used to track vitals, niacin doses, session cycles (exercise and sauna times), vitamins, and minerals for the 2-week program.

On page 179 is the *Detoxination Daily Report* used to track meals, niacin reactions and manifestations, symptomatic changes, and other metrics during the 2-week program. This form records three days per sheet, therefore, you will need to print several copies of the form to track your progress.

If you have opted in to the ***Get Detoxinated!***™ Program, then these two forms, once submitted, allow us to detect trends and health issues for statistical tracking. We are currently developing a mobile app for real-time monitoring, and subscribers will be automatically notified upon its release.

These forms and detailed instructions are found on our website at https://www.GetDetoxinated.com/book/.

DETOXINATION DAILY LOG

Client/Alias: _____ Age: _____ Sex: _____ Start Date: _____ End Date: _____

Niacin Target (10mg/kg): _____ of _____

THR Min/Max: _____ / _____   Beg. Fat%/BMI: _____ / _____   End Fat%/BMI: _____ / _____

Log Sheet #: _____

	PROGRAM DAY													
	1	2	3	4	5	6	7	8	9	10	11	12	13	14
Niacin Dose														
Hours of Sleep														
Blood Pressure	/	/	/	/	/	/	/	/	/	/	/	/	/	/
Weigh-In (lbs)														
Starting Body Temperature														
Start Time														
1st Cycle Exercise Time														
1st Cycle Sauna Time														
1st Sauna Temp (Highest Reached)														
1st Body Temperature														
2nd Cycle Exercise Time														
2nd Cycle Sauna Time														
2nd Sauna Temp (Highest Reached)														
2nd Body Temperature														
Stop Time														
Weigh-Out (lbs)														
Total Exercise Time														
Total Sauna Time														
Total Water Intake														
Oz of Cal-Mag Consumed														
Amount of Cell Salts Taken														
Amount of Potassium Taken														
Amount of Sodium Salts Taken														
Vitamin A Dose (IU)														
Vitamin B Complex Caps														
Vitamin B1 Dose (mg)														
Vitamin C Dose (mg)														
Vitamin D-3 Dose (IU)														
Vitamin E Dose (IU)														
Mineral Capsules														

Completed: Y / N   Continued on Next Daily Log: Y / N

© 2018 Sabre Hawk, LLC dba Detoxination Wellness Centers, Sacramento, CA

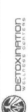

DETOXINATION WELLNESS CENTERS

DETOXINATION DAILY REPORT

Client/Alias: _____ Age: _____ Sex: _____ Start Date: _____ End Date: _____ Sauna Type: ☐convection ☐FIR

Log Sheet Page # _____ of _____

	Day:	Day:	Day:	Notes
PROGRAM DAY				
Diet:				
Breakfast				
Lunch				
Dinner				
Snacks				
Any particular cravings?				
Reaction to niacin				
Was there an increase or decrease?				
Did you take your supplements?	Y / N Notes:	Y / N Notes:	Y / N Notes:	
Since yesterday, any mental/physical experiences while away from the center?				
Gastrointestinal Status				
Did you experience any unusual feelings, thoughts, emotions, or physical manifestations during exercise or sauna therapy?				
Have there been any changes in any of your preprogram symptoms or conditions today? (Specify)				
Did you notice any new symptoms today? (Specify)				
Describe any improvements you notice today				

Completed: Y / N   Continued on Next Daily Log: Y / N

© 2017 · Sabre Hawk, LLC dba Detoxination Wellness Centers

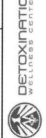

DETOXINATION
WELLNESS CENTERS

CONFIDENTIAL

Response Letter to the Medical Board of California

In 1986 a complaint was filed with the medical board against my father and HealthMed by four state physicians. The ensuing probe was later publicized in the Los Angeles Times. It was included in a Scientology hit piece denigrating the idea that someone like Hubbard, who holds the Guinness World Record for the most published works, could develop anything worthwhile.

Notice in the following excerpt from that article how the dangers of toxic body burden were largely unknown – or *minimized* – even as recent as the 1990s.

Los Angeles Times, *Scientology and Science* (Wednesday, 27 June 1990, page A1:1)

> ...In 1986, four doctors with the California Department of Health Services accused HealthMed of making "false medical claims" and of "taking advantage of the fears of workers and the public and about toxic chemicals and their potential health effects, including cancer." The doctors also criticized the foundation for supporting "scientifically questionable" research.
>
> The state physicians, who evaluate potential toxic hazards in the workplace, leveled the accusations in a letter that triggered an investigation by the state Board of Medical Quality Assurance. That probe was concluded last year without a finding of whether the detox treatment works.

Following is the 50-page response letter to the California Medical Board / Board of Quality Assurance which ended the investigation and preserved my father's medical license and career:

DAVID E. ROOT, M.D., M.P.H.

Diplomate, American Board of Preventive Medicine
Specializing in Occupational Medicine and General Practice

Board of Medical Quality Assurance
1430 Howe Avenue
Sacramento, CA 95825   January 7, 1987

Dear Dr. ██████:

    This letter is pursuant to a request by ████████████ and the
Board for information on the detoxification treatment of patients
showing signs and symptoms of toxic chemical exposure. ████████
indicated that you would be interested in the medical aspects of
this work.

    Interest in assessing the risks associated with human body
burdens of various toxic substances is growing throughout the world.
A number of agencies, including the World Health Organization and, in
this country, the National Institute for Environmental Health Sciences
are pursuing research objectives in this area, as are various
industries.

    As you are probably aware, this field can involve controversy.
Unfortunately, there have been a few individuals and groups who have
sought to incite and exploit public fears concerning chemicals in the
environment. Also, at times, quite legitimate public health concerns
from widely differing points of view have been aggressively debated in
the public arena.

    Therefore, the common frame of reference from which this subject
should be properly addressed is the peer-reviewed scientific
literature. Accordingly, I have prepared for you a comprehensive
review of the literature underlying this work and have included
extensive references.

    While this letter is quite long, it does not include all the
necessary information for a full study of the subject. Let me
therefore extend to you an invitation to visit my office if you wish
to further examine some of these matters.

    I have divided this review into five sections, a background
section, a review of signs and symptoms, a very brief look at the
assessment of xenobiotic exposure, detoxification methodology and
results. A separate addendum to this letter provides the noted
references.

One Scripps Drive • Suite 205 • Sacramento, California 95825 • (916) 924-9263

Page 2

I. HUMAN CONTAMINATION

     Concern about the storage of hazardous chemicals within the human body dates back several centuries and was formally examined as early as the 18th century by Ramazzini in his work on occupational diseases (1).

     From that time forward, exposure to chemicals has increased with an ever quickening pace. The largest expansion in the chemical revolution took place after World War II with a dramatic growth in the number and variety of hazardous chemicals which store in human tissues. As of 1980 over 400 chemicals had been identified in human tissue, some 48 in adipose tissue (2).

     The explosive post-war proliferation of toxic chemicals has left behind an enormous void of information on these substances, a vacuum which will require decades and tremendous human and financial resources to fill. The National Research Council reported in 1984 that almost no toxicity data is available for about 80% of the 50,000 odd chemicals now used commercially (3).

     This dearth of reliable data has in some instances placed the debate over the extent and significance of industrial and environmental chemical exposures on an emotional, rather than a scientific, footing. Charges and counter-charges are often exchanged in the absence of sound scientific investigation. While current legitimate public health concerns must be addressed, one must be mindful of the potential for the fraudulent exploitation of the public's fear of contaminants.

     Nevertheless, the potential health hazards associated with human body burdens of toxic chemicals are of increasing concern to private and governmental investigators throughout the world. The National Institute for Environmental Health Sciences, for example, has included among its research priorities the development of alternative designs for the standard cancer bioassay in order to make the end results more amenable to low-dose extrapolation. NIEHS has also called for the study of the metabolism and storage of PBB (polybrominated biphenyls) and possible means of reducing PBB body burdens (4).

     Human xenobiotic contamination takes place in many ways. There are exposures like the one in Michigan where people were contaminated by PBB through the dairy and beef food chain (5). These types of exposures affect large populations and have occurred in many nations. Their stories are legend in the environmental community and include dioxin in Seveso, Italy, PCB's in Japan and Taiwan, methyl isocyanate in Bhopal, India, and HCB's in Turkey (6-10). Taken together, over ten million people have been exposed around the world by these five incidents alone.

Accidental exposures also occur on a more narrow plane. A transformer may explode, exposing one or more persons to high concentrations of PCB's. Isolated industrial accidents may also bring about high body burdens of persistent toxicants.

Other forms of exposure are more pedestrian. In everyday life, workers and many others are routinely exposed to toxic substances. Whether it is caused by an overly zealous pesticide applicator, the inhalation of gasoline fumes containing benzene and lead or chronic occupational exposures, contamination by toxic substances is a common occurrence in modern society. Even infants receive a chemical legacy from their mothers during gestation as well as while feeding at their breasts (11, 12). The practical result of these common low level exposures is increases in human body burdens with age, because many chemicals accumulate in bone and fat much more rapidly than the body can excrete them.

Substance Abuse

The abuse of drugs and medicines provides yet another source of increasing xenobiotic body burdens. Based upon statistics compiled by the National Institute on Drug Abuse (13), over 50 million people in the nation have used such fat-soluble drugs as cocaine, phencyclidine (the street drug called PCP or angel dust), diazepam or THC, the major active chemical in marijuana. As might be expected, standard analytical methods are now being developed to accurately determine adipose tissue levels of these substances in humans. Even now, however, there are a great many studies which suggest that these drugs do store for prolonged periods.

A. Cocaine

With regard to cocaine, Nayak (14) deduced that the binding of lipophilic cocaine to tissue may play a more important role in determining its overall pharmacokinetics than its plasma protein binding capacity. Comparing acutely and chronically exposed rats, Nayak (14) has shown that cocaine concentrations from six hours to four weeks after injection were much higher in fat than concentrations in other tissues of chronically treated animals.

Page 4

Norcocaine, another cocaine metabolite, was observed in rat brain (16). It has been shown to be a pharmacologically active metabolite of cocaine in the brain of dogs (15), monkeys (17), and rats (16) and is oxidized to its highly reactive nitroxide free radical This, in conjunction with the prolonged storage of cocaine in the fat of the chronically exposed, may explain the systemic toxicity of cocaine.

When combined with an understanding of the potential for mobilization of fat stored chemicals; this animal data suggests that the sequestration of cocaine and metabolites in fat depots of the chronically exposed individual can be expected to produce a slow prolonged release of cocaine into the plasma long after discontinuation of drug use. The result is the potential for long-term unpredictable adverse effects in humans due to either slow or rapid releases of fat stored residuals.

B. Diazepam

In studying Diazepam (DZ), DeSilva (19) found that single oral doses of DZ produced low and rapidly declining DZ blood levels. Repeated doses caused a progressive increase of DZ levels. The major metabolite of DZ, N-desmethyldiazepam (DMDZ) (18), appeared 24-36 hours after the first dose and thereafter the levels increased rapidly, approaching those of DZ levels. Upon discontinuing the drug, DZ and DMDZ disappeared from the blood very slowly, detectable levels of DMDZ persisting longer than DZ.

Those blood level fall-off patterns indicate a rapid and extensive uptake by tissues, followed by slow redistribution in the blood of DZ and DMDZ. As it is highly lipophilic, DZ is likely to be stored in adipose tissue, being released during lipolysis or under other conditions which promote mobilization. In addition, DZ was found in high concentrations in the fat of rats two hours after I.P. doses of 0.6 mg/kg (20). Marcucci (21) stated that it was clear from the results in his study that DZ accumulates in the adipose tissue in relatively high concentrations in mice, rats and man.

C. Phencyclidine

With regard to phencyclidine, James (22) concluded that tissue distribution of phencyclidine in the rat correlated well with its high lipid solubility. The drug shows a strong affinity for adipose tissue, and high levels persist long after the drug has cleared from the blood.

Page 5

Misra (23) demonstrated the persistence of PCP and its metabolites for prolonged periods in brain and adipose tissue of rats. Due to the high lipid solubility of PCP, its tissue levels greatly exceeded the plasma levels.

In Martin's study on mice (24), three days after PCP administration the only detectable levels of PCP were in fat. Chronic exposure resulted in elevated levels of PCP in fat up to 21 days.

Misra feels that "the long sojourn of PCP in the adipose tissue and relatively slow egress therefrom explains cumulative effects upon multiple dosing and raises the possibility of the mobilization or release of large amounts of the drug from fat stores in situations involving food deprivation, marked weight loss or stress" (23).

D. Tetrahydrocannabinol

The plant Cannabis Sativa, from which marijuana is derived, contains at least 421 individual components, of which 61 are specific to cannabis. Ten are now routinely quantified when identifying cannabis samples (25).

Several animal studies document long-term storage of cannabinoids in fat and lipid containing tissues after Delta-8 and Delta-9-Tetrahydrocannabinol (THC) administration (26-30).

Kennedy (27), using the whole body autoradiography of the pregnant mouse and administration of labelled THC, found high concentrations of radioactivity in fat and a few organs. Kreuz (28) reported a ten-fold greater THC accumulation in fat of rats compared with other tissues. And Agurele (31), studying the metabolism of labelled THC in rabbits, found high levels of radioactivity in the fat of the rabbit three days after administration. As might be expected, repeated doses of THC lead to accumulation in fat (28). At least one study has documented the presence of THC in human adipose tissue (32).

The Significance of Human Contamination

If harmful fat-soluble chemicals moved into the major fat stores of the body and remained in place, perhaps there would be less cause to worry about human body burdens. However, these chemicals do not stay put, nor do they go only to relatively unimportant fat deposits.

Page 6

Whenever lipids move into the blood, so too do the chemicals stored
in them (33). This occurs every day as part of the normal functioning
of the body. For example, the evening fast (while sleeping at night),
aerobic exercise, and common emotional stress mobilize fat and hence
stored chemicals (34,35,36).

Once in the blood these chemicals have the opportunity to reach
every part of the body. For some chemicals this means they will be
broken down into components, for example, by reaction in the liver.
The components may go back to the fat or, if they are water soluble, may
be excreted. However, many of the chemicals industry has created do not
metabolize easily. They were developed so that they would not break down.

A good example are the polychlorinated biphenyls (PCB's). These
chemicals were made for use in high temperature environments and
withstand even moderately hot fires. In 1968, an outbreak of an
epidemic occurred in Yusho, Japan that was traced to the contamination
of cooking oil by PCB's. This material has been shown to store in
body fat. Under normal conditions, very little, if any, of this
material is excreted.

Complaints of PCB intoxication are usually reported as fatigue,
headache and digestive disorders. Women occasionally complain of
menstrual disorders. There may be a productive cough and some
numbness in the extremities (37). Abnormalities in babies from
mothers exposed to PCB from Yusho oil during pregnancy have been
widely reported (38).

The clinical features were dark brown pigmentation of mucus
membranes and skin, gingival hyperplasia with pigmentation, a tendency
for babies to be born small for their due date, eruption of teeth at
birth, hypersecretion of the meibomian gland and edema of the orbital
area. Babies continued to be born with these features for some time
after the exposure demonstrating that the developing fetus is a major
excretory pathway for women of childbearing age.

Animal experimentation demonstrated that the principal areas
affected by long term exposure to PCB's at low levels are the
lymphatic system, liver and gastrointestinal tract (39).

It has subsequently been shown that people with high level exposure
to PCB's have clinically identifiable effects related to their immune
system (40).

The body is equipped to excrete water soluble chemicals, but is
not as well developed to excrete the fat soluble ones. Therefore, if
the body cannot break these chemicals down into excretable
metabolites, they tend to redistribute into the various fatty portions

of the body. In addition to the adipose tissue lying just below the skin layers of the body, the brain, the sheathing of the nervous system, and the liver are also major fat depots. Persistent human contaminants are routinely found in these depots (2). Distribution is fairly even; recent studies by Ryan, et al, as well as the Centers for Disease Control, of cadaver burdens of 2,3,7,8-TCDD (dioxin) found comparable levels in each of the adipose depots examined with the exception of heart adipose tissue, where levels were lower (41,42).

The effects from chemicals which store in the body are not always easy to describe. First, there is inadequate health data on the vast majority of the 50,000 chemicals in commercial production (3). What data does exist tends to reflect effects in rodents rather than humans, and is nearly always the result of large exposures to a single chemical. It is difficult, if not impossible, to estimate the effects of chemical mixtures, and there have been very few such tests in animals. In addition, animal tests are notoriously poor at indicating the potential for effect on the skin or the nervous system.

There are also a number of individual and environmental variables which modulate the effects of xenobiotic contamination in humans. Individual variables include:

* Genetic susceptibility or predisposition (43)
* Age (44,45)
* Nutritional status (46,47)
* Lifestyle habits, such as alcohol and cigarette consumption (48-52)
* Biochemical uniqueness as it relates to the efficiency of metabolic pathways for absorption, uptake into tissues and excretion, and the degree of affinity of certain target tissues for xenobiotics in the body (53)
* The presence and degree of psychosocial stresses (54)
* The absense or presence of pre-existing disease.

Environmental variables include:

* Degree of exposure
* Duration of exposure
* The specific chemicals entering the body
* The interreactions of chemicals inside the body (55):
  Synergistic (combined effect greater than the sum of the
      effects of the individual agents);
  Potentiating (one component enhancing the effects of another);
  Additive (combined effect is the sum of the effects of the
      individual agents);
  Antagonistic (combined effect is less than the sum of the
      effects of the individual agents).
* The latent period between exposure and effect (56).

Page 8

The basis for most human data comes from study of populations exposed in the work place or in large scale exposures such as those previously mentioned. There are usually a wide number of effects, some which may be unique to the chemicals in question, but most of which certainly are not.

Health effects associated with chemical exposure are characterized by a hierarchy of events. Figure 1, developed by Colucci, indicates the relative frequency of the different health effects associated with chemical exposure (57). This scale of effect severity is continuous up to the point of death. Morbidities are usually defined by clinical and sub-clinical signs. These are changes at the system level, the organ level, or the cellular level. They are generally measurable quantitatively, but may be directly observable by a clinician in a qualitative manner.

Morbidity due to chemical body burdens may take the form, for example, of increased blood pressure, decreases in numbers of red blood cells, increases in white blood cells, increases in specific enzymes, decreases in the rate of nerve impulse transmission, rashes, joint swelling and pain, IQ and personality trait change, and a myriad of other clearly observable effects, all considered adverse.

Below morbidity are the subtle effects of chemical exposure. Over a decade ago Golberg defined the study of these effects as "subliminal toxicology" (58). More often than not, these effects are observable as subtle functional changes such as slowing of motor reactions, impaired regulation of appetite, reduced visual discrimination capacities, fatigue, and memory loss. Mello reports that "the early and incipient stages of (these) intoxications are marked by vagueness and ambiguity" (59). These symptoms pose a special problem for health professionals. Weiss and Simon point out, "these are not deficits that induce people to seek out physicians" (60).

The significance of chemical exposure is not that low level exposures can cause subtle symptoms. Rather it is that such symptoms are the sentinels of possibly more serious chemical-related disease. Underlying toxicology research is the time tested model of biological action which suggests that the greater the chemical exposure, the greater the resultant effect. This model has been found to hold true for chemical health threats such as those now found in environmental and occupational settings. In the most common cases of chronic intoxication, clinical tests are frequently negative, despite the clear and plainly undesirable symptomatology (61). However, as body burdens rise, so too do concentrations in the blood, and resulting exposures in vital organ systems.

Page 9

It comes as little suprise, therefore, to find a progression to
more serious disease states with increasing body burdens. Figure 2
presents this progression in humans exposed to polychlorinated and
polybrominated biphenyls (PCB's& PBB's).

The significance of increasing chemical body burdens comes from
the increased probability of chronic disease, whether subtle or
acutely manifest.

FIGURE I

Spectrum of Biological Response to Pollutant Exposure (57)

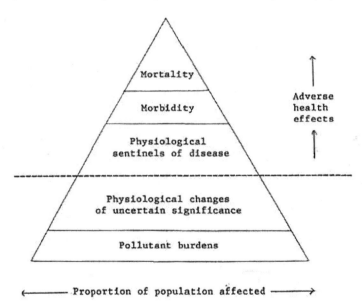

Figure II
The Progression of Disease Associated with
Bioaccumulation of Polyhalogenated Biphenyls

EXPOSURE	BIOACCUMULATION*		HEALTH INDICATORS	BIOLOGICAL RESPONSE
Ambient 35 yrs	.03 ppb. Blood PBB	(73)	None Observed	Normal
	.004 ppm fat PBB	(80)		
	2.3 ppb blood PB	(107)		
Low-level or Ambient 35 yrs	11 ppb blood PBB	(64)	Subtle Symptoms	Fatigue (64,79)
	.4 ppb fat PBB	(137)		Headache
				Muscle weakness
	5 ppb blood PCB	(115,125)		Nervousness
				Joint pain
				(See Table of Symptoms)
Occupationa or Extended Low-Level	90 ppb blood PBB	(62)	Subclinical and Clinical Signs	Immune dysfunction (64)
	25 ppm fat PBB	(137)		Elevated DEA titer (62)
	44 ppb blood PCB	(79)		levated SGOT- SGPT (64.70)
Extended Occupationa	603 ppb blood PBB	(136)	Overt Signs and Symptoms	Dermal (79,107) abnormalities
	196 ppm fat PBB	(136)		Abdominal pain
	356 ppb blood PCB			Eye irritation
Massive	13-75 ppm fat PCB	(84)	Premature Death	Major Systemic failures (84)
Lifelong Ambient Exposure	8.7 ppm fat pcb	(124)	Premature Death	Cancer (124)
	5.1 ppm fat DDT			

* Fat concentrations measured on a per lipid weight bases.

Page 11

II. SIGNS AND SYMPTOMS

From a review of the literature, one can tabulate a pattern of signs and symptoms associated with xenobiotic contamination (63-143). Depending upon the nature and seriousness of a given exposure, these manifestations may be quite severe or subtle. Subtle signs and symptoms, as noted previously, may represent early warning markers of more serious chemically related disease. The tabulation which follows provides some indication of the scope of xenobiotic activity as identified in the literature to date.

CARDIOVASCULAR

Hypertension
Irregular heart beat
Chest pain and tightness
Myocardial infarction

OPTHALMIC

Eye irritation
Dimness of sight (amblyopia)
Double vision (diplopia)
Blurred vision
Eye oscillation (nystagmus)
Abnormal pupil reactions

NEUROLOGICAL

These can be categorized into various subsets, as follows:

Nervous system arousal problems

- lethargy
- depression
- nervousness
- irritability
- emotional instability
- photophobia
- sleeplessness
- sleepiness

Associative

- decreased mental acuity
- impaired memory
- confusion
- disorientation
- slowed functional adolescent impairment

Physiological/Metabolic

- headaches
- emotional instability
- loss of appetite
- irritability
- fatigue

Sensory

- vision impairment
- hearing impairment
- perception changes (taste/smell)
- burning sensation
- paresthesias
- hallucinations

Motor

- speech impairment
- muscle weakness
- tremors
- difficulty walking
- seizures
- incoordination and clumsiness
- dizziness

Peripheral neuropathies

RESPIRATORY

Wheezing or difficulty in breathing
dryness of the nose and throat
chest tightness
nasal obstruction/congestion
coughing
chest pain (pleuritic)

DERMATOLOGICAL

    Urticaria
    acne
    rash
    darkening or thickening
    discoloration or deformity of nails dryness
    sun sensitivity

GASTROINTESTINAL

    nausea
    vomiting
    abdominal pain
    abdominal cramps
    diarrhea

MUSCULOSKELETAL

    Joint pain
    Swollen joints
    myalgia

IMMUNE SYSTEM

    Overactivity (allergies)

        - Rhinitis
        - Urticaria
        - Alergic contact dermatitis
        - Bronchial asthma
        - Arthralgia (autoimmunity)

    Underactivity

        - Impaired host resistance

HEPATIC

    jaundice
    hepatomegaly

Page 14

As one reviews these symptoms, it is possible to cross-categorize. For instance, the symptoms of fatigue and lethargy, in addition to being manifestations of neurological dysfunction, may be indications of a generalized metabolic dysfunction due to the possible deleterious effects of xenobiotics on intra-cellular tissue respiratory pathways (144,145). However, they may also be indications of having completed a hard day's work. Therefore, it is essential to note that persons exposed to toxic chemicals often complain of a constellation of symptoms (58,63); moreover, several studies have shown that the existing differences between exposed groups and control groups could not otherwise be explained without considering the etiologic role for exposure to toxic substances (53,93,98).

III. ASSESSMENT OF XENOBIOTIC EXPOSURE

The diagnosis of disease in an individual is generally based upon a clinical history and physical examination. The physician may then use additional information, including laboratory determinations (e.g., blood, urine and adipose tests) and more specialized procedures (e.g., radiological examinations and biopsies) in developing a possible diagnosis. Specific laboratory tests and exposure history questionnaires can be of value when they are critically interpreted. Exposure history questionnaires should be quite detailed in order to elicit complete information (including incidents a patient may not have recognized as exposure related) and should examine the work, home and general environments.

Correct interpretation of laboratory results requires knowledge of the accuracy and precision of the test, and the normal range of values found in healthy people.

In a review such as this it is not possible to adequately treat a topic as broad in scope as the diagnosis of chemically related ills. There are a great many tests available which could be used to assess organ and system functions. In arriving at a diagnosis, one would select, of course, those which are most appropriate based upon the observations and information to hand, including the known or suspected chemical agent to which an individual has been exposed. While the literature on this matter is voluminous, a good summary has been compiled by a scientific panel organized by the Board of Directors of Universities Associated for Research and Education in Pathology (146).

Page 15

The following is an overview of tests which may be used to assess organ and system functions as they relate to chemical toxicity.

1. Liver function (147,148)

    (i)   aspartate aminotransferase AST (SGOT)

    (ii)   Alanine inotransferase, ACT (SGPT)

    (iii)   gamma-glutamyl transpepsiase (GGTP

    (iv)   alkaline phosphatase

    (v)   bilirubin

    (vi)   Serum bile acids

2. Renal function (149-152)

    (i)   Urinary specific gravity

    (ii)   pH

    (iii)   proteinuria

    (iv)   BUN and serum creatinine levels

    (v)   glomerular filtration rate

    (vi)   renal enzyme activities

3. Reproductive function (153-155)

    (i)   Sperm assays

            Semen physiology can be assessed by evaluating: a) count
            (density), b) motility, c) morphology (cytology), and d) YYF
            test (representative of Y-chromosome nondisjunction during
            spermatogenesis) (156).

            Factors such as age, smoking and medication need to be taken
            into consideration when interpreting the results from such
            studies (157).

    (ii)   Ovarian and uterine function assays

Page 16

4. Immunologic function (158-160)

    (i)   white blood cell count and differential

   (ii)   B cell and T cell counts (lymphocytes)

  (iii)   T-lymphocyte activation tests

  (iv)   T4/T8 ratios (T cell differential counts)

   (v)   Serum Immunoglobulin screen

  (vi)   Serum complement levels.

5. Lung function (161)

    (i)   FVC

   (ii)   FEVI

  (iii)   Residual volume/total lung capacity ratio

  (iv)   Alveolar diffusion capacity

6. Opthalmic function (162)

    (i)   visual acuity

   (ii)   visual field determinations. These may be of value in assessing low grade xenobiotic toxicity.

7. Nervous System (163-185)

    (i)   Electrophysiological techniques to measure:

        a) Sensory nerve conduction velocity
        b) motor nerve conduction velocity
        c) electromyographic examination (may be used to assess peripheral nerve dysfunction)
        d) sensory loss

   (ii) EEG -may be useful in assessing latent or abnormal electrical activity in the brain as a result of xenobiotic exposure.

(iii) a) I.Q. tests (e.g., Wechsler Adult Intelligence Scale) and
other tests to assess memory.

b) Personality profile evaluation or psychometric testing
(e.g., Minnesota Multiphasic Inventory)

c) Perceptual-motor skill assessments, if used correctly
and with objectivity give a baseline of nervous system
integrity.

d) Other standardized neurobehavioral and psychological
tests (memory, problem solving, etc.).

Tests of blood, urine, adipose tissue or other organ tissues can,
of course, also be carried out to directly assess xenobiotic body
burdens. The above organ and system function tests are best carried
out in company with such direct assays. A great deal more work is
needed in this area, however, as our analytical capabilities have been
far outstripped by the rapid proliferation of new chemical compounds.

IV. DETOXIFICATION METHODOLOGY

While we still do not fully understand the bio-active mechanisms
or the pharmacokinetics of many toxic substances, physicians have
known for centuries that health problems can ensue as a result of body
burden accumulations of xenobiotics and have looked for ways to safely
and effectively reduce body burdens.

Ramazzini, in his landmark 1713 work, Diseases of Workers, notes
that writers of works on poisons at that time "advise; in general,
remedies that have the power of setting the spirits and blood mass in
motion and of provoking sweat" (1), a recommendation which seems at
once simplistic and yet profound in light of what is now known, nearly
275 years later, concerning the pharmacokinetics and metabolism of foreign
compounds.

Any procedure to reduce body burdens of lipophilic toxins must
satisfy three essential requirements:

Page 18

1. Enhanced mobilization of the stored chemical from lipid reservoirs.

2. Adequate distribution of mobilized chemicals to the portals of excretion.

3. Enhanced routes of excretion. Routes of excretion include:

> hepatic
> gastrointestinal
> renal
> skin: via sweat and/or sebum

From these fundamentals, an effective regimen for reducing body burdens of xenobiotics would consist of the following elements:

1. Enhanced mobilization of xenobiotics from lipophilic sites.

To enhance the mobilization of lipophilic chemicals, one has to find ways of increasing lipid turnover. By increasing mobilization, one can then free the stored xenobiotic into the circulation (176).

Factors that increase lipid mobilization include:

A. Exercise.

Numerous studies have demonstrated that exercise can increase the mobilization of lipids, and that the rate of mobilization is dependent upon rate of blood flow through the adipose tissue (177-190).

The energy requirements of exercising muscle are met by the oxidation of both fat and carbohydrate. For example, by 40 minutes of continuous exercise, plasma lipid (free fatty acid, FFA) contributes approximately 37% and plasma glucose 27% to muscle oxidative metabolism as assessed by the uptake of oxygen by leg muscles (191).

B. Nicotinic Acid (Niacin)

This vitamin, in high doses, has profound antilipolytic effects and has been used in the treatment of hyperlipidoemias. Nicotinic acid, however, blocks the mobilization of FFA from adipose tissue to the blood for only a short time, approximately 30 to 90 minutes depending upon dose. This effect is followed by a pronounced rebound and overshoot of FFA in the blood (192-199).

Page 19

C. Polyunsaturated oils

Several studies have shown that polyunsaturated fat feeding can bring about significant changes in body fat composition. Polyunsaturated oils have been found to replace existing adipose tissue stores, thereby mobilizing some lipids, as in a lipid exchange mechanism (200-203).

Mobilization of persistent fat-stored xenobiotics into the blood now permits their excretion through the various excretory pathways. If one only mobilizes these chemicals without enhancing their excretion on there would be distribution of them to other tissue sites, such as the muscle compartment, with consequent redistribution back to the lipid areas.

It is theoretically unwise therefore to increase the mobilization of xenobiotics without ensuring their enhanced excretion. However, when utilizing the methodology described herein, analysis of blood concentrations of contaminants during treatment has shown that excretion keeps pace with the levels of xenobiotics mobilized from fat stores (204).

2. Increasing Circulation

Improving blood flow and cardiovascular efficiency will permit two things:

A. Increased blood flow through the adipose tissue, thereby enhancing the "pickup" of mobilized xenobiotics;

B. Increasing blood flow to the skin thereby enhancing xenobiotic elimination through sweat and sebum.

Three factors which would play a role in this are:

* the use of aerobic exercise, which enhances cardiac output and peripheral blood flow to adipose tissue and the epidermis;

* the use of heat stress, which increases circulation (205,206).

* the use of nicotinic acid which is a potent vasodilator (207, 208). Its effect seems to be largely dependent upon increased release of prostaglandins E2, a potent vasodilator, from the vascular wall. Its impact upon peripheral blood flow is at its greatest as the levels of nicotinic acid are rising in the blood (209).

Page 20

3.   Enhancing Routes of Excretion

A. Hepatic Function

The liver contains enzyme systems that biochemically transform lipophilic xenobiotic compounds into more water soluble derivatives. These polar derivatives can then be excreted by the kidneys (210-214), or into the bile (the production of which is enhanced by polyunsaturated oils, 215-217), and from there to the gastrointestinal tract and feces. This mixed-function oxidase (MFO) system is inducible, i.e., its activity levels can be increased. Factors that induce the hepatic MFO system are:

* elevations in the concentration of certain environmental chemicals such as DDT and other halogenated hydrocarbon insecticides, PCB's, urea herbicides, polycyclic hydrocarbons, the dioxins and chlorinated aromatic hydrocarbons (218).

* drugs (not used in the methodology described herein), such as phenobarbital (219),

It is evident therefore that increased lipid mobilization of xenobiotics will increase the xenobiotic load to the liver and thereby induce MFO system activation and this will enhance excretion.

B. Overcoming enterohepatic recirculation.

Various means have been suggested to overcome enterohepatic recirculation. Cholestyramine, high fiber diets, vegetable diets, sucrose polyester and paraffin have all been used (220-224). Each has a side effect which tends to stress the liver due to fat deposition. A less stressing approach to overcoming enterohepatic circulation is the use of dietary polyunsaturated oil. Total fecal steroid excretion has been increased by 45 percent through use of corn oil versus cocoa butter as the source of dietary fats (201). This type of supplement has been found to produce a decrease in plasma cholesterol which appears to be indicative of increased fecal excretion (214, 225).

Associated with overcoming enterohepatic recirculation is the potential for a lowering of absorption of important nutrients and thus increasing the toxicity of persistent chemicals such as PCB's and PBB's (226). This can be especially important for the lipophilic vitamins. Vitamin A, for example, undergoes extensive enterohepatic recirculation and must be supplemented at higher than normal doses if increased fecal excretion is likely (215). This is particularly important for PCB poisonings where animal studies show a significant decrease of vitamin A in the liver and serum during PCB administration thus leading to an increased A requirement (227,228).

Page 21

Another essential vitamin supplement is ascorbic acid. It has been found, for example, that PCB contamination brings about a depression in the activities of the enzymes L-gluconolactone oxidase and dehydroascorbatase along with an increased urinary excretion of L-ascorbic acid. PCB toxicity disturbs the normal histological pattern of the liver cells and also significantly changes the hepatic lipid composition. L-ascorbic acid supplementation can afford protection against the enzyme activity alterations and histological changes resulting from PCB toxicity (229).

C. Renal excretion.

This depends on the efficiency of hepatic MFO system to conjugate and make more water soluble the derivatives from the nonpolar chemicals.

D. Epidermal excretion

This is a potential major pathway whereby toxic chemicals can be excreted, either via the sweat or sebum. Not only does increased heat exposure increase sweat production, but sebum also. Both sebum (230-239) and sweat (240-249) can act as routes of excretion for xenobiotics, including organohalides (233, 250, 251) and heavy metals (241-243, 248). During epidermal excretion, of course, one must ensure adequate intake of water and appropriate salts as well as nutritional supplements to ensure the body does not become depleted.

V. CLINICAL SUMMARY

A.   Safety.

The utilization of a methodology such as that outlined above has been accomplished safely and effectively and reports have appeared in the literature (250-254). The origin of the technique is somewhat unique in that it was developed by a non-physician, the late L. Ron Hubbard, who concluded in the early 1970's that residues of drugs and other contaminants stored in the adipose and set about developing a means of reducing body burdens. In the late 1970's the method began to be used by a number of drug rehabilitation facilities internationally.

Page 22

While this demonstrated clearly the safety of the regimen,
it was not until 1981 that physicians and environmental scientists
began to look into the efficacy of the technique in addressing body
burdens of some of the most persistent halogenated hydrocarbons.
They found the method not only well grounded in the traditional
literature, but surprisingly effective in reducing body burdens of
toxicants previously thought to be more. or less permanently stored in
fat tissue. The results of these studies led to the utilization of
the method by physicians in the U.S. and abroad, beginning in the
early 1980's.

In California, my associates and I have treated approximately
1,300 individuals over the past 5 years. Referrals for treatment are
predominantly from physicians and other professionals. A number of
industries and insurers have been encouraged by the return to work
following treatment of persons who had previously been on disability.

An initial study of the regimen on 103 individuals found it to be
very well tolerated (252). Of course, such a program would be
inadvisable for pregnant women, persons with coronary artery disease
or certain other major physical disabilties.

With respect to the mobilization of xenobiotics from fat depots
it has been suggested that such might result in elevated blood levels.
However, as was noted previously, analysis of chemical concentrations
in the blood during treatment indicates that excretion of body burdens
keeps pace with mobilization from fat stores (251). In other words,
there was no significant elevation of blood levels of toxicants during
treatment.

B.   Body Burden Reductions

Preliminary studies of this regimen have found it to bring about
significant body burden reductions of several compounds examined,
including the highly persistent PCB's and PBB's. A study by Schnare,
et al, of Michigan farmers exposed to PBB examined 16 organohalides,
including PCB and PBB congeners and three pesticides (250). 13 were
present in lower concentrations at post-treatment sampling. Seven of
the 13 reductions were statistically significant; reductions ranged
from 3.5 to 47.2 percent, with a mean reduction among the 16 chemicals
of 21.3 percent (s.d. 17.1 percent).

A gathering of physicians, toxicologists and researchers from the
Mt. Sinai School of Medicine, Wayne State University, Battelle
Laboratories and several other institutions and governmental agencies
examined these preliminary findings and made recommendations which
included a four month follow-up adipose biopsy of those treated. This
follow-up analysis was completed and showed a reduction in all 16
chemicals averaging 42.4 percent (s.d. 17.1 percent)and ranging from
10.1 to 65.9 percent. Ten of the 16 reductions were statistically

Page 23

significant. Thus, a continuing reduction of body burdens following treatment was clearly demonstrated.

In 1983, Roehm made a similar observation during treatment of a Vietnam veteran with a history of exposure to dioxin and DDE, a persistent metabolite of the now-banned pesticide, DDT (254). Adipose levels of DDE were determined using mass spectrometry pre-treatment and at four intervals post treatment. After 250 days DDE was determined to be 97% removed.

A more recent study examined PCB and HCB (hexachlorobenzene) congeners in electrical workers paired by age, sex and PCB exposure potential and divided into treatment and control groups (251). Both groups maintained their normal work routines during the treatment and follow-up periods. Adjusted for reexposure as represented in the control group, HCB body burdens were reduced by 30% at post-treatment and 28% at three months post-treatment. Mean reduction of PCB cogeners was 16% at post-treatment and 14% at three months post-treatment. Analysis of variance indicates these reductions are statistically significant ($F < .001$).

A great many individual case histories have demonstrated the efficacy of this method in reducing body burdens of certain organohalides. A capacitor factory worker, for example, with an extremely high PCB adipose tissue level of 102 ppm was recently treated. Post-treatment level was 37 ppm, a 65% reduction (255).

C.   Symptom remission.

The achievement of body burden reductions might be of less importance if reversible symptoms were not relieved concurrently. Clinical observations noted in the literature and by physicians who have applied this methodology, however, suggest it brings about a significant improvement in signs and symptomatology. One study examined 120 individuals referred for treatment of health effects which diagnostic assessment suggested were due to chemical exposure (253). This patient population was selected to replicate the age and sex distribution of the population examined by Anderson, et al (64). Symptoms examined were based upon 15 health effects studied by Anderson in a PBB-exposed population and an unexposed control population from rural Wisconsin. The symptom prevalence in the pre-treatment group was comparable to Anderson's chemically exposed population, while symptom prevalence in the post-treatment group was significantly reduced and comparable to that identified in Anderson's unexposed control group (Figure 3).

A similar study was recently completed on 21 patients with known heavy exposures to contaminants such as pesticides, fungicides,

Page 24

FIGURE 3

Symptom Prevalence of Chemically Exposed and Unexposed Reference
Populations and a Chemically Exposed Treatment Group

Symptom	Chemically Exposed Population (Anderson)	Healthy Population (Anderson)	Treatment Group (pre-treatment)	Treatment Group (post-treat.)	
					1
Rash	17 %	9 %	18 %	4 %	**
Acne	12	5	16	4	*
Skin Thickening	9	3	9	4	
Paresthesis	19	5	14	2	**
Weakness	13	3	16	4	*
Uncoordination	21	5	7	0	*
Diziness	20	3	18	2	**
Fatigue	52	15	79	5	**
Nervousness	22	2	14	4	*
Disorientation	6	0	11	0	**
Headaches	41	14	40	9	**
Joint Pain	43	23	5	0	*
Muscle Pain	23	8	42	5	**
Abdominal Pain	13	7	33	11	**
Constipation	6	2	26	2	**

1. The difference in symptom prevalence after treatment is significant at the
following levels: $*$ = $p < 0.05$; $**$ = $p < 0.01$.

solvents and PCB's. Statistical analyses were performed to determine the effects of this treatment on symptom severity. The analyses found a highly significant decrease in severity following treatment.

It is noteworthy that many of those who had been treated for severe chemical exposure had been in a diseased state for several months or years prior to treatment and had been examined and treated by several physicians, with little to no relief of signs and symptoms.

A 54 year-old woman, for example, was treated for heavy exposure to pesticides (256). Exposure had taken place approximately 5 years prior to treatment. In 1980, a neurologist determined her health problems to be chemically caused. Over the next 5 years she sought out a variety of physicians with no significant change in her health status. In 1986 adipose tissue levels of DDE were measured at 38 ppm with DDT at 4.8 ppm. Adipose heptachlor epoxide was measured at 33 ppm. Total PCB's were at 20 ppm. Following treatment, adipose DDE dropped to 3.5 ppm, DDT to .6 ppm, heptachlor expoxide to 1.2 ppm and total PCB's to 2.0 ppm. Alleviation of signs and symptoms was dramatic. Physicians have reported numerous similar case histories.

It should be noted that the initial study of this method (252) found that patients with high blood pressure had a mean reduction of 30.8 mm systolic, 23.3 mm diastolic. Cholesterol level mean reduction was 19.5 mg/100 ml, while triglycerides did not change. These findings of blood pressure and cholesterol level reduction have been confirmed over the past 4 years in the treatment of over 1,300 patients.

D.   Significant decrease in drug, alcohol and tobacco consumption.

With regard to both discontinuance of substance abuse and body burden reductions, this detoxification methodology has been shown to be of considerable value. Body burden reduction data is limited due to limited analytical capabilities for adipose tissue. However, an adipose reduction in four subjects of approximately 50 percent of both THC and its hydroxy-metabolite was seen following 21 days of treatment (257). In one other case, PCP was identified in the urine of a police narcotics officer undergoing treatment 3 years after a bottle of concentrated liquid PCP was thrown into his face (258).

In examining alcoholism, a recent study by Laposata and Lange is of interest (259). They note that acetaldehyde, the end product of oxidative ethanol metabolism, contributes to alcohol-induced disease in the liver, but cannot account for damage in organs such as the pancreas, heart, or brain, where oxidative metabolism is minimal or absent; nor can it account for the varied patterns of organ damage

Page 26

found in chronic alcoholics. They observed that many human organs metabolize ethanol through a nonoxidative pathway to form fatty acid ethyl esters. Organs lacking oxidative alcohol metabolism yet frequently damaged by ethanol abuse had high fatty acid ethyl ester synthetic activities and showed substantial transient accumulations of fatty acid ethyl esters. The fact that there may be an ethanol metabolite which stores in human tissues is worthy of further investigation.

With regard to substance abuse, a statistical analysis was recently completed of 204 patients who had used drugs, alcohol and/or tobacco prior to this particular detoxification treatment (260). Patients rated their use of these substances before and after treatment on a scale of 1 to 5 (light to heavy). The mean and median age of the patients was 34. Statistical analysis showed that using this treatment methodology, probability of improvement for drugs was 98 percent, for alcohol, 91 percent and for tobacco, 68 percent.

Of the 109 patients who had used so-called "recreational" drugs, all but 6 discontinued drug use following treatment and these 6 reduced drug use. 30 of these patients had rated their drug use as heavy (5 on the scale) and all of these discontinued drug use following treatment. Of the 16 patients who rated their alcohol use as heavy, 13 discontinued alcohol consumption following treatment.

E.   Future studies.

While this methodology certainly provides sound and safe treatment for chemical exposures, the data reported on to date suggest several avenues for further work. A more detailed study of a larger cohort should be undertaken. There are, additionally, several compounds (the dioxins, for example) for which body burden reductions have not as yet been adequately studied. There is also a considerable variation in the percentage of reduction noted for the various organohalide congeners which have been studied. This is not well understood.

Several studies have found that a continuing reduction in body burdens takes place after treatment is terminated. An understanding of this phenomenon will require more extensive research on mobilization and excretion pathways.

The fact that symptom remission has been seen to accompany reductions of body burdens is encouraging. As there is a known progression of disease associated with the bioaccumulation of xenobiotics, it is likely that achieving substantial reductions of

Page 27

such body burdens may lessen the risk of future disease and improve, overall, the health status of the individual. Such a detoxification methodology as is described above thus may prove an important addition to those tools available to the physician in assisting patients to cope with those chronic health problems which often follow serious chemical exposures.

Yours truly,

David E. Root, M.D., M.P.H.

Encl: References
    cc: ████████████ , Esq.

Page 28

REFERENCES

1.   Ramazzini, B., Diseases of Workers (1713), New York Academy
      of Medicine, History of Medicine Series, Vol. 28, Hafner
      Publishing Co., New York, 1964.

2.   U.S. Environmental Protection Agency. Chemicals identified
      in human biological media, a data base. US EPA. Washington,
      D.C. EPA 560/13-80-036B, PB81-161-176, 1980.

3.   National Research Council, Toxicity Testing: Strategies to
      Determine Needs and Priorities, National Academy of Sciences
      Washington, D.C., 1984.

4.   National Institutes of Health, NIH Guide for Grants and Con-
      tracts, Vol. 12, No. 7, July 15, 1983.

5.   Anderson, J.W., Woolf, M.S. and Lilis, R. Symptoms and
      clinical abnormalities following ingestion of polybrominated
      biphenyl-contaminated food products. Ann. N.Y. Acad. Sci.
      320:684-702, 1979.

6.   Santi, L., Boeri, R., Remotti, G., Ideo, G., Marni, E.,
      Puccinelli, V. Five Years After Seveso, Lancet, Feb 6, 1982,
      1(8267):343-344, 1982.

7.   Inamura, M., Tung, T. A trial of fasting cure for PCB-poi-
      soned patients in Taiwan. Am. J. Ind. Med. 5:147-153, 1984.

8.   Masuda, Y., Yoshimura, H., Polybrominated biphenyls and
      dibenzofurans in patients with Yusho and their toxicological
      significance: a review, Am. J. Ind. Med. 5(1-2):31-44, 1984.

9.   Andersson, N., Kerr Muir, M., Salmon, A.G., Wells, C.J.,
      Brown, R.B., Purnell, C.J., Mittal, P.C., Mehra, V., Bhopal
      disaster: eye follow-up and analytical chemistry. Lancet,
      March 30, 1985, 1(8431)761-762., 1985.

10.   Peters, H.A., et al., Epidemiology of hexachlorobenzene
      induced porphyria in Turkey. Arch. Neurol. 39:744, 1982.

11.   Schwartz, P.M., Jacobson, S.W., Fein, G., Jacobson, J.L.
      Price, H.A. Lake Michigan fish consumption as a source of
      polychlorinated biphenyls in human cord serum, maternal
      serum and milk. Am. J. Publ. Health 73:293-296, 1983.

12.   Wolff, M.S., Occupationally Derived Chemicals in Breast Milk,
      Am. J. of Indus. Med. 4:259-281, 1983.

Page 29

13.   National Institute on Drug Abuse, Washington, D.C., National
        Household Survey on Drug Abuse, 1985.

14.   P.K. Nayak, A.L. Misra, S.J. Mule: Physiological disposition
        and biotransformation   of (H) cocaine in acutely and
        chronically treated rats. J. Pharmacal. Exper. Ther. 196,
        556-569 (1976).

15.   L.A. Woods, F.G. McMahon, M.H. Seevers: Distribution and
        metabolism of cocaine in the dog and rabbit. J. Pharm. Exp.
        Ther. 101, 200-204 (1951).

16.   A.L. Misra, P.K. Nayak, M.N. Phtel, N.L. Vadlamani, S.J.
        Mule: Identification of norcocaine as a metabolite of (H)-
        cocaine in rat brain. Experimentia 30, 1312-1314 (1974).

17.   R.L. Hawks, I.J. Kopin, R.W. Colburn, N.B. Thoa: Norcocaine:
        A pharmacologically active metabolite of cocaine found in
        brain. Life c Sci. 15, 2189-2195 (1974).

18.   A.J. DeSilva, B.A. Koechlin, G. Bader: blood level
        distribution patterns of diazepam and its major metabolite
        in man. J. Pharm. Sci. 55, 692-702 (1966).

19. R.L. Foltz, A.F. Ferrtiman, R.B. Foltz: Diazepam and its
        major metabolite, N-desmethyldiazepam in "GC/MS assays for
        abused drugs in body fluids" (Ed. R.L. Filtz, A.F. Fentiman
        and R.B. Foltz) pp. 128-149. National Institute on Drug
        Abuse (NIDA) Research Monograph Series 32, 1980.

20.   M.A. Schwartz, B.A. Koechlin, E. Postman, S. Palmer, G.
        Krol: Metabolism of diazepam in rat, dog and man. J. Pharma-
        cal. Exp. Ther. 149, 423-435 (1965).

21.   F. Marcucci, R. Fanelli, M. Frova, P.L. Morselli: Levels of
        diazepam in adipose tissue of rats, mice and man. Eur. J.
        Pharmacol. 4, 464-466 (1968).

22.   S.H. James, S.H. Schnoll: Phencyclidine: Tissue distribution
        in the rat. Clin. Toxicol. 9, 573-582 (1976).

23.   A.L. Misra, R.B. Pontani, J.G. Bartolomeo: Persistence of
        phencyclidine (PCP) and metabolites in brain and adipose
        tissue and implications for long-lasting behavioral effects.
        Res. Commun. in Chern. Pathol. Pharmacol. 24, 431-445 (1979).

24.   B.R. Martin: Long-term disposition of phencyclidine in mice.
        Drug Met. Dispos. 10, 189-193 (1982).

Page 30

25.   C.E. Turner: Chemistry and metabolism in "Marihuana
        Research Findings: 1980" (Ed. R.C. Peterson) pp. 81-97.
        National Institute on Drug Abuse Research Monograph Series
        31, 1980.

26.   S. Agurell, I.M. Milsson, A. Ohlson, F. Sandberg: On the
        metabolism of tritium-labelled delta-1-tetrahydrocannabinol
        in rabbit. Biochem. Pharmacal. 19, 1333-1339 (1970).

27.   B.T. Ho, G.E. Fritchie, P.M Kralik, L.F. Englert, W.M.
        Mcisaac, J. Idanpaan-Heikkila: Distribution of tritiated-1-
        delta-9-tetrahydrocannabinolin   rat   tissues   after
        inhalation.J. Pharm. Pharmacol. 22, 538-539 (1970).

28.   J.S. Kennedy, W.J. Waddell: Whole-body autoradiography of
        the pregnant mouse after administration of C-delta-nine-
        THC. Toxicol. Appl. Pharmacol. 2, 252-258 (1972).

29.   D.S. Kreuz, J. Axelrod: Delta-9-tetrahydrocannabinol:
        Localization in body fat. Science 179, 391-393 (1973).

30.   B. Mantilla-Plata, R.D. Harbison: Distribution studies of (
        C) delta-9-tetrahydrocannabinol in mice: Effect of vehicle,
        route of administration, and duration of treatment.
        Toxicol. Appl. Pharmacal. 34, 292-300 (1975).

31.   A. Ohlsson, J-E. Lingren, A. Wahlen, S. Agurell, L.E.
        Hollister,   H.K.   Gillespie: Plasma   delta-9-
        tetrahydrocannabinol concentrations and clinical effects
        after oral and intravenous administration and smoking.
        Clin. Pharmacal. Ther. 28, 409-416 (1980).

32.   Fdn for Adv. in Science and Ed., "THC Research Update",
        Research Bulletin (1983).

33.   Findlay, G.M. and De Freitas, A.S.W, DDT movement from adi-
        pocyte to muscle cells during lipid utilization. Nature 229:
        63, 1971.

34.   Schlierf, G. and Dorow E. Diurnal patterns of triglycerides,
        free fatty acids, blood surgar, and insulin during carbohy-
        drate-induction in man and their modification by nocturnal
        suppression of lipolysis. J. Clinic. Invest. 52:732, 1973.

35.   Wirth A., Schlierf G., and Schettler, G. Physical Activity
        and lipid metabolism. Wochenschir. 57:1195, 1979.

Page 31

36. Cleghorn, J. Psychosocial influences on a metabolic process: The psychophysiology of lipid mobilization. Canad. Psychiat. Ass. J. 15:539-546, 1970.

37. Koda, H., and Masuda, Y., Relation between PCB levels in the blood and clinical symptoms of Yusho patients, Fukuoka Acta Med. 66(10): 624-628, 1975.

38. Yoshimura, T., Epidemiological study on Yusho babies born to mothers who had consumed oil contaminated with polychlorinated biphenyls, Fukuoka Acta Med. 65(1): 74-80, 1974.

39. Kimbrough, R.D., Squire, R.A., Linder, R.E., et al, Induction of liver tumours in rats by polychlorinated biphenyl (Aroclor 1254), J. Natl. Cancer Inst., December, 1975.

40. Loose, L.D., Pittman, K.A., Benitez, K.F., Silkworth, J.B., Polychlorinated biphenyl and hexachlorobenzene induced humoral immunosuppression, J. Reticuloendothel Soc. 22(3):253-71,1977.

41. Ryan, J.J., Williams, D.J., American Chemical Society Meeting, Washington, D.C., 1983.

42. Needham, Larry, Centers for Disease Control, Atlanta, Personal communication, 1986, regarding study soon to be published in Chemosphere.

43. Auerbach, A.D.; Wolman, S.R., Susceptibility of Fanconi's anaemia fibroblasts to chromosome damage by carcinogens. Nature 261:494-496. 1976.

44. Grice, H.C.; Burek, J.D.; editors. Age-associated (geriatric) pathology: its impact on long-term toxicity studies. In: Grice, H.C., ed. Current issues in toxicology. New York: Springer-Verlag: p. 51-117, 1984.

45. Van Duuren, B.L., Smith, A.C., Melchionne, S.M., Effect of aging in two-stage carcinogenesis on mouse skin with phorbol myristate acetate as promoting agent. Cancer Res. 38:865-866. 1978.

46. Crosby, D.G. , The nonmetabolic decomposition of pesticides. Ann. N.Y. Acad. Sci. 160:82-96. 1969.

47. Searle, C.E., editor. Chemical Carcinogens. ACS monograph 173. Washington, D.C.: American Chemical Society. 788p. 1976.

Page 32

48.   Ferguson, R.K., Vernon, R.J., Trichloroethylene in combina-
        tion with CNS drugs. Effects on visual-motor tests. Arch.
        Environ. Health 20:462-467, 1970.

49.   Windemuller, F.J.B., Ettema, J.H., Effects of combined
        exposures to trichloroethylene and alcohol on mental capacity,
        Int. Arch. Occup. Environ. Health 41:77-85.

50.   U.S. Dept. of H.E.W., Office on Smoking and Health,
        Introduction and summary. In: The Office. Smoking and
        Health: a report of the Surgeon .General. DHEW Publication
        no.(PHS)79-50066. Washington D.C.: U.S. Dept. of H.E.W.,
        Public Health Service, p. 1.1-1.35, 1979.

51.   U.S. Dept. of H.E.W., National Institute for Occupational
        Safety and Health. Interaction between smoking and occupation-
        al exposures. In: The Department, Office on Smoking and Health.
        Smoking and health: a report of the Surgeon General.
        Washington, D.C.: U.S. Dept. of H.E.W., Public Health Service,
        p. 7.1-7.25. 1979.

52.   Selikoff, I.J., Hammond, E.C., Churg, J., Asbestos exposure,
        smoking and neoplasia, J. Am. Med. Assoc. 204:104-112. 1968.

53.   Calabrese, E.J., Principles of animal extrapolation. New
        York: John Wiley & Sons. 603p. 1983.

54.   Cleghorn, J. Psychosocial influences on a metabolic process:
        The psychophysiology of lipid mobilization. Canad. Psychiat.
        Ass. J. 15:539-546, 1970.

55.   Fairchild, E.J., Concepts of effects of combined exposures
        to chemicals. In: Andrzejewski, S.W.; Tarkowski, S.; eds.
        Health effects of combined exposures to chemicals in work and
        community environments: proceedings of a course, October
        18-22, 1983, Lodz, Poland. European Cooperation on Environ-
        mental Health Aspects of the Control of Chemicals: interim
        document 11. Copenhagen: World Health Organization, Regional
        Office for Europe. p. 15-43.

56.   Corn, M., Breysse, P.N., Review of "Working List of Issues to
        be Addressed in a Finding of Completeness," Prepared for
        the Maryland State Hazardous Waste Facilities Siting Board by
        the Department of Environmental Health Sciences, School of
        Hygiene and Public Health, The Johns Hopkins University. 29p.
        1983. Available from: The Board, Annapolis, MD.

Page 33

57.   Colucci, A.V., Hammer, D.I., Williams, M.E., et. al. Pollutant Burdens and Biological Response. Arch. Environ. Health 27:151-154, 1973.

58.   Goldberg, L. Safety of Environmental Chemicals - The Need and the Challenge. Fd. Cosmet. Toxicology 10:523-529, 1972.

59.   Mello, N.K.   Behavioral toxicology: A developing discipline. Fed. Proc. 34(9):1832-1834, 1975.

60.   Weiss, B. and Simon, W. Quantitative perspectives on the long term toxicity of methylmercury and similar poisons. In Weiss, B. and Laties, V.G. (eds) Behavioral Toxicology. Appleton-Century-Crofts, New York, 1976.

61.   Scharnweber, H.C., Spears, G.N., Cowles, S.R.   Chronic Methyl chloride intoxication in six industrial workers. J. Occup. Med. 16:112, 1974.

62.   Anderson, H.A., Wolff, M.S., Fischbein, A., et.al. Investigation of the Health Status of Michigan Chemical Corporaton Employees. Environ. Health Perspec. 23:187-191. 1978.

63.   Anderson, H.A., Lilis, R., Selikof, I.J., et.al. Unanticipated Prevalence of Symptoms Among Dairy Farmers in Michigan and Wisconsin. Environ. Health Perspect. 23:217-226. 1978.

64.   Anderson, H.A., Wolff, M.S., Lilis, R., et.al. Symptoms and Clinical Abnormalities Following Ingestion of Polybrominated Biphenyl-Contaminated Food Products. Ann. N.Y. Acad. Sci. 320:684-702. 1979.

65.   Bekesi, J.G., et al. Impaired Immune Function and Identification of PBB in Blood Compartments of Exposed Michigan Dairy Farmers and Chemical Workers. Drug and Chern. Tox. 2:179-191. 1979.

66.   Bencko, V., Symon, K. Test of Environmental Exposure to Arsenic and Hearing Changes in Exposed Children. Environ. Health Perspect. 19:95-101. 1977.

67.   Bornschein, R., Pearson, D. Reiter, L. Behavioral Effects of Moderate Lead Exposure in Children and Animal Models: Parts CRC Crit. Rev. Tox. 8(1&2):43 & 101. 1980.

68.   Bryce-Smith, D. Behavioral effects of lead and other heavy metal pollutants. Chern. Br. 8:240. 1972.

Page 34

69. Catton, M.J. Subclinical neuropathy in lead workers.   Br.
     Med. J. 2:80-82. 1970

70. Cavanagh, J.B. Peripheral Neuropathy Caused by   Chemical
     Agents. CRC Crit. Rev. Tox. 2(3):365. 1974.

71. Cheek, L. An Insurance Perspective on Proposals for Hazard-
     ous Substance Compensation. Conference jon Liability and
     Compensation for Injuries and Damage Caused by Release of
     Hazardous Waste. California Foundation on the Environment
     and the Economy. Sacramento, CA. 29 Nov 1983.

72. Colucci, A.V., Hammer, D.I., Williams, M.E., et al. Pollu-
     tant   Burdens and Biological Response. Arch. Environ. Health
     27:151-154. 1973.

73. Dale, W.E., Curley, A., Cueto, C. Hexane Extractable Chlori-
     nated Insecticides in Human Blood. Life Sci. 5:47. 1966.

74. Damstra, T. Environmental chemicals and nervous system dys-
     function. Yale J. Biol. Med. 51:457. 1978.

75. Dews, P.B. Epistemology of screening for behavioral toxici-
     ty. Environ. Health Perspect. 26:37. 1978.

76. Eckardt, R. E., Industrial intoxications which may simulate
     ethyl alcohol intake. Ind. Med. Surg. 40:33. 1971.

77. Elkins, H.B. Maximum acceptable concentrations, a comparison
     in Russia and the United States. AMA Arch. Environ. Health
     2:45. 1961.

78. Evans, H.L., Weiss, B. Behavioral toxicology. Contemporary
     Research in Behavioral Pharmacology. Blackman, D.E., Snager,
     D.J., Eds. Plenum Press. New York. 1978. p 449

79. Fischbein, A. Wolff, M.S., Lilis, R., et.al. Clinical Find-
     ings Among PCB-exposed Capacitor Manufacturing Workers. Ann.
     N.Y. Acad. Sci. 320:703-715. 1979.

80. Frankon, J.J., Luyton, B.J. Comparison of Dieldrin, Lindane
     and DDT Extractions from Serum and Gas-Liquid Chromatography
     using Glass Capillary Columns. J. Assoc. Offic. Anal. Chern.
     59(6):1279-1284. 1976.

81. Fullerton, P.M. Industrial disease of the central nervous
     system. Soc. Occup. Med. Trans. 19:91. 1969.

Page 35

82.   Furchtgott, R. Behavioral Effects of Ionizing Radiations. Psychological Bulletin 60(2):157-199. 1963

83.   Golberg, L. Safety of Environmental Chemcals -- The Need and the Challenge. Fd. Cosmet. Toxicol. 10:523-529. 1972.

84.   Goto, M., Higuchi, K. The symptomatology of Yusho. Fukuoka Acta Med. 60:409-431. 1969.

85.   Hansen, H., Weaver, N.K., Venable, F.S. Methyl chloride intoxication. Arch. Ind. Hyg. Occup. Med. 8:328. 1953.

86.   Hewitt, W.L. Clinical implicatons of the presence of drug residues in food. Fed. Proc. 34(2):202-204. 1975

87.   Higuchi, K., Ed. PB poisoning and pollution. Kidansha, Tokyo and Academic Press, New York. 1976.

88.   Isbister, J.L. The short-term effects of PBB on health. Michigan Department of Public Health report, Feb. 23, 1977.

89.   Johnstone, R. T. Clinical inorganic lead intoxication. Arch. Environ. Health. 8:250. 1964.

90.   Kegal, A.H., McNally, W.C., Pope, A.S. Methyl chloride poisoning from domestic refrigerators. J.A.M.A. 93:353. 1929.

91.   Kimbrough, R.D. The toxicity of polychlorinatd polycyclic compounds and related chemicals. CRC Crit. Rev. Toxicol. 2:445-498. 1974.

92.   Kolata, G.B. Behavioral Teratology: Birth Defects of the Mind. Science 202:732-734. 1978

93.   Kuratsune, M., Masuda, Y., Nagayama, J. Some recent findings concerning Yusho. National Conference on Polychlorinated Biphenyls, Proceedings. USEPA 560-6-75-004. Office of Toxic Substances, Washington, D.C.: 14-29. 1976.

94.   Kuratsune, M., Morikawa, Y., Hirohata, T., et al. An epidemiological study on "Yusho" or chlorobiphenyls poisoning. Fukuoka Acta Med. 60:513. 1969.

95.   Lilis, R. Behavioral effects of occupational carbon disulfide exposure. In Behavioral Toxicology, Early Detection of Occupational Hazards. C. Xintaras, B. Johnson and I deGroot, Eds.:51-59. H.E.W. Publication No. (NIOSH)74-126. 1974

Page 36

96.   Lilis, R., Anderson, H.A., Valciukas, J.A., et.al. Compari-
       son of findings among residents on Michigan dairy farms and
       consumers of produce purchased from these farms. Environ.
       Health Perspect. 23:105-110. 1978.

97.   MacDonald, J.D.C. Methyl chloride intoxication: report of 8
       cases. J. Occup. Med. 6:81. 1964.

98.   Meester, W.D., and McCoy, D.J. Human Toxicology of polybro-
       minated biphenyls. Paper presented at Symposium on Environ-
       mental Toxicology, Seattle, Washington. Aug. 4. 1976.

99.   Mello, N.K. Behavioral toxicology: A developing discipline.
       Fed. Proc. 34(9):1832-1834. 1975

100.   Metcalf, D.R., Holmes, J.H. EEG, Psychological, and Neurolo-
       gical Altrratons in Humans with Organophosphorus Exposure.
       Ann. N.Y. Acad. Sci. 160:357-365. 1969.

101.   Mitchell, C.L., Tilson, H.A. Behavioral Toxicology in Risk
       Assessment: Problems and Research Needs. CRC Crit. Rev. Tox.
       9:265-274. 1982.

102.   Mitchell, C.L. Assessment of neurobehavioral toxicity: prob-
       lems and research needs. Trends in Pharmacological Sciences.
       4:195-198. 1983

103.   Moore, L.S., Fleischman, A.I. Subclinical Lead Toxicity. J.
       Orthomolec. Psychiat. 4:61070. 1975.

104.   Nebert, D.W., Elashoff, J.D., Wilcox, K.R. Possible Effect
       of Neonatal Polybrominated Biphenyl Exposure on the Develop-
       mental Abilities of Children. Am. J. Pub. Health. 73(3):286-
       289. 1983.

105.   National Academy of Sciences. Airborne Lead in Perspective.
       Committee on Biologic Effects of Atmospheric Pollutants. NAS
       Washington, D.C. p 50. 1972.

106.   Norton, s. Is behavior or morphology a more sensitive indi-
       cator of central nervous system toxicity? Environ. Health
       Perspect. 26:21. 1978

107.   Ouw, H.K., Simpson, G.R., Siyali, D.S. Use and Health Ef-
       fects of Aroclor 1242, a Polychlorinated Biphenyl, in an
       Electrical Industry. Arch. Envr. Health 31:189-194. 1976.

108.   Reiter, L. Neurotoxicology -- meet the real world. Neuro
       behav. . Toxicol 2:73. 1980.

109.   Repko, J.D., Corum, C.R. Critical Review and Evaluation of
        the Neurological and Behavioral Sequelae of Inorganic Lead
        Adsorption. CRC Crit. Rev. Tox. 6(2):135. 1979.

110.   Repko, J.D., Lasley, S.M. Behavioral, Neurological, and
        Toxic Effects of Methyl Chloride: A Review of the Litera-
        ture. CRC Crit. Rev. Tox. 6(4):283-?. 1979.

111.   Ruffin, J.B. Functional testing for behavioral toxicity: a
        missing dimension in experimental environmental toxicology.
        J. Occup. Med. 5:117. 1963.

112.   Scharnweber, H.C., Spears, G.N., Cowles, S.R. Chronic methyl
        chloride intoxication in six industrial workers. J. Occup.
        Med. 16:112. 1974.

113.   Schnare, D.W., Denk, G., Shields, M., et.al. Evaluation of a
        Detoxification Regimen for Fat Stored Xenobiotics. Med. Hyp.
        9:265-282. 1982.

114.   Schnare, D.W., Ben, M., Robinson, P.C., et.al. Reduction of
        Human Organohalide Body Burdens - Final Research Report.
        Foundation for Advancements in Science and Education. Los
        Angeles. July 1983.

115.   Schnare, D.W., Robinson, P.K., Reduction of Hexachloro-
        benzene and Polychlorinated Biphenyl Human Body Burdens,
        World Health Organization, International Agency for Research
        on Cancer Scientific Publications Series, Vol. 77, Oxford
        University Press, In Press.

116.   Seagull, E. Developmental abilities of children exposed to
        polybrominated biphenyls. Am. J. Pub. Health 73:281-285.
        1982.

117.   Seppalalinen A.M., Hernberg S. Sensitive technique for de-
        tecting subclinical lead neuropathy. Br. J. Ind. Med.
        29:443-449. 1972.

118.   Seppalainen, A.M., Toal, S., Hernberg. S., et al. Subclini-
        cal Neuropathy at 'Safe' Levels of Lead Exposure. Arch
        Environ. Health 30:180-183. 1975

119.   Smrek, A., Needham, L. Simplified clean-up procedures for
        adipose tissue containing polychlorinated biphenyls, DDT and
        DDT metabolites. Bull. Environ. Contam. Toxicol. 28:718-722.
        1982.

Page 38

120.   Spyker, J.M., Sparber, S.B., Goldberg, A.M. Subtle conse-
        quences of methylmercury exposure: Behavioral deviations in
        offspring of treated mothers. Science 177:621. 1972.

121.   Spyker, J.M., Chang, L.W. Delayed effects of prenatal expo-
        sure to methylmercury: brain ultrastructure and behavior.
        Teratology 9:A37. 1974

122.   Spyker, J.M. Behavioral teratology and toxicology. In Beha-
        vioral Toxicology. Eds. Weiss, B. Laties, B.G. Plenum, New
        York. p311-344. 1976.

123.   Spyker, J.M. Assessing the impact of low level chemicals on
        development: Behavioral and latent effects. Fed. Proc.
        34(9):1835. 1975.

124.   Unger, M., Olsen, J. Organochlorine compounds in the adipose
        tissue of deceased people with and without cancer. Envr.
        Res. 23:257-263. 1980.

125.   US EPA. Chemial Contaminants in Nonoccupatonally Exposed US
        Residents. EPA-600/1-80-001. USEPA, Washington, D.C. 1980.

126.   Valciukas, J.A., Lilis, R., Wolff, M.S., et al. Comparative
        neurobehavioural study of a polybrominated biphenyl-exposed
        population in Michigan and a nonexposed group in Wisconsin.
        Environ. Health Perspect. 23:199-210. 1978.

127.   Valciukas, J.A., Lilis, R. Eisinger, J., et al. Behavioral
        indicators of lead neurotoxicity: Results of a clinical
        field survey. Int. Arch. Occup. Environ. Health 41:217-236.
        1978.

128.   Valciukas, J.A., Lilis, R., Anderson, H.A., et al. The
        neurotoxicity of polybrominated biphenyls: Results of a
        Medical Field Survey. Ann. N.Y. Acad. Sci. 320:357-366.
        1979.

129.   Valciukas, J.A., et al. Central nervous system dysfunction
        due to lead exposure, in press.

130.   Weiss, B., Simon, w. Quantitative perspectives on the long
        term toxicity of methylmercury and similar poisons. In
        Weiss, B., Laties, V.G. (eds.) Behavioral Toxicology. New
        York. Appleton-Century-Crofts. 1976.

131.   Weiss, B., Spyker, J.M. Behavioral Implications of Prenatal
        and Early Postnatal Exposure to Chemical Pollutants. Pedia-
        trics 53(5.II):851-859. 1974.

Page 39

132. Weiss, B., Brozek, J. Hanson, H. et al. Effects on behavior, Chap. X. In: The Evaluation of Chemicals for Societal Use. Ed. N. Nelson. Washington, D.C. National Academy of Sciences. 1974.

133. Weiss, B., Brozek, J. Hanson, H. et al. Effects on behavior. Principles for Evaluating Chemicals in the Environment. NAS 1975.

134. Weiss, B. Specifying the Nonspecific. USSR-US Workshop on Behavioral Toxicology, Suzdal, Russia. Nov. 1978.

135. Weiss, B., Laties, V.G. Assays for behavioral toxicity: a strategy for the Environmental Protection Agency. Test Methods for Definition of Effects of Toxic Substances on Behavior and Neuromotor Function. 1(suppl. 1):213. Neurobehavioral Toxicology. 1979. (Eds. Geller, L., Stebbins, W.C., Wayner, M.J.)

136. Wolff, M.S., Anderson, H.A., Camper, F., et al. Analysis of adipose tissue and serum from PBB exposed workers. J. Environ. Path. Tox. 2:1397-1411. 1979.

137. Wolff, M.S., Anderson, H.A., Selikoff, I.J. human tissue burdens of halogenated aromatic chemicals in Michigan. JAMA 247(15):211-2116. 1982.

138. Zavon, M.R. Problems in recognition of lead intoxication. Arch. Environ. Health 8:262.   1964.

139. Kreiss, K., Zack, M. Kimbrough, R.D., et al., Association of Blood Pressure and Polychlorinated Biphenyl Levels, J.A.M.A. 245:2505, 1981.

140. Kerfoot, E.J., Mooney, T.F., Formaldehyde and Paraformaldehyde Study in Funeral Homes, Am. Indust. Hygiene Assoc. Jrnl., July, 1975.

141. Sioris, L.J., Krenzelok, E.P., Phencyclidine intoxication: A literature review, Am. J. Hosp. Pharm 35:1362-1367, 1978.

142. Baker, E.L., Peterson, W.A., Holtz, J.L., et al., Subacute Cadmium Intoxication in Jewelry Workers: - An Evaluation of Diagnostic Procedures, Archives of Environmental Health, May/ June, 1979.

143. Harada, M., Congenital Minamata Disease: Intrauterine Methylmercury Poisoning, Teratology 18:285-288, 1978.

Page 40

144.   Luckey, T.D., Venugopal, B., Metal Toxicity in Mammals. I. Physiologic and chemical basis for metal toxicity. New York Plenum Press, 1977.

145.   Clarkson, T.W., Factors involved in heavy metal poisoning. Fed. Proc. 36:1634-1639, 1977.

146.   Grisham, J.W., ed., Health Aspects of the Disposal of Waste Chemicals, Chapter 4, Assessment of Health Effects, Pergamon Press, New York, 1986.

147.   Price, C. P., Alberti, K.G.M.M., Biochemical assessment of liver function. In: Write, R., Alberti, K.G.M.M., Karran, S., Millward-Sadler, G.H., eds. Liver and biliary disease. New York: W.B. Saunders Company. p. 381-416.

148.   Guzelian, P.S., Research needs for hepatic injury due to environmental agents. Environ. Health Perspect. 48:65-71.

149.   Wedeen, R. P., Toxic wastes and kidney disease: research needs. Environ. Health Perspect. 48:73-76.

150.   Kluwe, W.M., Hook, J.B., Effects of environmental chemicals on kidney metabolism and function. Kidney Int. 18:648-655.

151.   Hook, J.B., Serbia, V.C., Potentiation of the action of nephrotoxic agents by environmental contaminants. In: Porter, G.A., ed.   Nephrotoxic mechanisms of drugs and environmental toxins. New York: Plenum Medical Book Co. p. 345-356.

152.   McCormack, K.M., Kluwe, W.M., Rickert, D.E., Sanger, V.L., Hook, J.B., Renal and hepatic microsomal enzyme stimulation and renal function following three months of dietary exposure to polybrominated biphenyls. Toxicol. Appl. Pharmacol. 44:539-553.

153.   U.S. Department of Energy, Oak Ridge National Laboratory. Assessment of risks to human reproduction and to development of the human conceptus from exposure to environmental substances. Proceedings of U.S. Environmental Protection Agency-Sponsored Conferences: October 1-3, 1980, Atlanta, GA, and December 7-10, 1980, St. Louis, MO. ORNL/EIS-197. EPA-600/9-82-001. Oak Ridge, TN: The Laboratory. 152p.

154.   Dixon, L., Symposium on target organ toxicity: gonads (reproductive and genetic toxicity). Cosponsored by Society of Toxicology and National Institute of Environmental Health Sciences, December 1-4, 1976, Vanderbilt University, Nashville, TN. Environ. Health Perspectives. 24.

155. Mattison, D.R., Ross, G.T., Oogenesis and ovulation. In: Vouk, V.B., Sheehan, P.J., eds. Methods for assessing the effects of chemicals on reproductive functions. New York: John Wiley & Sons, Inc., p. 17-22.

156. Wyrobek, A.J., Methods for evaluating the effects of environmental chemicals on human sperm production. Environ. Health Perspec. 48:53-59; 1983.

157. Bloom, A.D., editor. Guidelines for studies of human populations exposed to mutagenic and reproductive hazards: proceedings of conference held Jan. 26-27, in Washington, D.C. White Plains, NY: March of Dimes Birth Defects Foundation. 163p.

158. Spreafico, F., Vecchi, A., Immunomodulation by xenobiotics: the open field of immunotoxicology. In: Fudenberg, H.H., Whittem, H. D., Ambrogi, F., eds. Immunomodulation. New frontiers and advances. Proceedings of a symposium on reent advances on immunomodulators, May 14-16, Viareggio, Italy, New York: Plenum Press p. 311-329, 1984.

159. Bekesi, J.G., Selikoff, I.J., Altered immune function in Michigan dairy farmers and chemical workers exposed to polybrominated biphenyls. In: Asher, I.M., ed. Inadvertent modification of the immune response: the effects of foods, drugs and environmental contaminants. Proceedings of the Fourth FDA Science Symposium, Aug. 28-30, 1978, Annapolis, MD. U.S. Dept. of Health and. Human Services, Food and Drug Administration, p. 210-212.

160. Dean, J.H., Luster, M.I., Boorman, G.A., Lauer, L.D., Procedures available to examine the immunotoxicity of chemicals and drugs. Pharmacal. Rev. 34:137-148.

161. Shigematsu, N., Ishimaru, s., et al., Respiratory Involvement in Polychlorinated Biphenyls Poisoning, Environmental Res. 16:92-100, 1978.

162. Seppalainen, A.M., Raitta, C., Huuskonen, M.S., N-Hexane induced changes in visual evoked potentials and electroretinograms of industrial workers. Electroencephalogr. Clin. Neurophysiol. 47: 492-498.

163. Schaumberg, H.H., Markowitz, L.S., Arezzo, J.C., Monitoring Potential neurotoxic effects of hazardous waste disposal. Environ. Health Perspect. 48:61-64.

Page 42

164.   Schaumber, H.H., Spencer, P.S., Toxic models of certain disor-
        ders of the nervous system - a teaching monograph. Neurotoxicol.
        1:209-220, 1979.

165.   Landrigan, P.J., Baker, E.L., Feldman, R.G., et al., Increased
        lead absorption with anemia and slowed nerve conduction in child-
        ren near a lead smelter. J. Pediatr. 89:904-910.

166.   Arezzo, J.C., Schaumberg, H.H, Vaughn, H.G., et al., Hind limb
        somatosensory evoked potentials in the monkey: the effects of
        distal axonopathy. Ann. Neurol. 12:24-32, 1982.

167.   Seppalainen, A.M., Harkonen, H., Neurophysiological findings
        among workers occupational exposed to styrene. Scand. J. Work
        Environ. Health 3:140-146, 1976.

168.   Seppalainen, A.M., Lindstrom, K., Martelin, T., Neurophysiologi-
        cal and psychological picture of solvent poisoning. Am. J. Ind.
        Med. 1:31-42, 1980.

169.   Arezzo, J.C., Schaumburg, H.H., Use of the "Optacon" as a screen-
        ing device: a new technique for detecting sensory loss in
        individuals exposed to neurotoxins. J. Occup. Med. 22:461-464,
        1980.

170.   Arezzo, J.C., Schaumberg, H.H., Peterson, C.A., Rapid screening
        for peripheral neurophathy: a field study with the "Optacon".
        Neurology 33:626-629.

171.   Aminoff, M.J., Peripheral sympathetic function in patients with a
        polyneuropathy. J. Neurol. Sci. 44:213-219, 1980.

172.   Damstra, T, Environmental chemicals and nervous system dysfunc-
        tion. Yale J. Biol. Med. 51:457-468, 1978.

173.   Landrigan, P.J., Toxic exposures and psychiatric disease -
        lessons from the epidemiology of cancer. Acta Psychiatr. Scand.
        67 Suppl. 303:6-15, 1983.

174.   Brown, G.G., Preisan, R.C., Anderson, M.D., et al., Memory per-
        formance of chemicals workers exposed to polybrominated
        biphenyls. Science 212:1413-1415, 1981.

175.   Baker, E.L., Letz, R., Fidler, A, A Computer-Administered
        Neurobehavioral Evaluation System for Occupational and Environ-
        mental Epidemiology, J. Occupational Me. 27(3): 206-212, 1985.

176.   Findlay, G.M., DeFreitas, A.S.W., DDT movement from adipocyte to
        muscle cell during lipid utilization, Nature 229:63, 1971.

177.   Wirth, A., Schlierf, G., Schetler, G., Physical activity and li-
       pid metabolism. Klin. Wochenshri. 57:1195, 1979.

178.   Norris, B., Schade, D.S., and Eaton, R.P., Effects of altered
       free fatty acid mobilization on the metabolic response to
       exercise. J. Clin. Endoc. Met. 46:254, 1978.

179.   Ahlborg, G., Felig, P., Hagenfeldt, L., Hendler, R., and Wahren,
       J., Splanchnic and Leg Metabolism of Glucose, Free Fatty Acids,
       and Amino Acids. Journal of Clinical Investigation 53:1080-1090
       1974.

180.   Taylor, A.W., Shoemann, D.W., Lovlin, R. and Lee, S., Plasma
       free fatty acid mobilization with graded exercise. J. Sports
       Med. 11:234-240, 1971.

181.   Klein, Von H.J., Kubicek, F. and Spiel, R., Lipid Metabolism in
       Coronary Patients During Physical Exercise. Weiner klinische
       Wochenschrift 86:543-546, 1974.

182.   Friedberg, S.J., Harlan, Jr., W.R, Trout, D.L., Estes, Jr.
       E.H., The Effect of Exercise on the Concentration and Turnover
       of Plasma Nonesterfied Fatty Acids. J. Clin. Invest. 39:215,
       1960.

183.   Oscai, L.R. and Holloszy, John O., Effects of Weight Changes
       Produced by Exercise, Food Restriction, or Overeating on Body
       Composition. Journal of Clinical Investigation 48:2124-2128
       (1969).

184.   Friedberg, S.J., Sher, P.B., Bogdonoff, M.D. and Estes, Jr.,
       E.H., The dynamics of plasma free fatty acid metablism during
       exercise. J. Lipid Research 4:34-38 (1963).

185.   Carlson, L.A. and Pernow, B., Studies on blood lipids during
       exercise. Journal of Laboratory and Clinical Medicine 58:
       673-681 (1961).

186.   Gollnick, P.D. Free Fatty Acid Turnover and the Availability
       of Substrates as a :Limiting Factor in Prolonged Exercise
       Ann. N.Y. Acad. Sci. 301:64-71 (1977)

187.   Taylor, A.W., The Effects of Different Feeding Regimens and
       Endurance Exercise Programs on Carbohydrate and Lipid Metabol-
       ism. Canadian J. of Applied Sport Sciences 4:2:126-130 (1979).

188.   Bulow, J., Adipose tissue blood flow during exercise. Danish
       Medical Bulletin 30:2:85-100 (1983).

Page 44

189.   Cobb, L.A., Ripley, H.S., Jones, J.W., Free Fatty Acid Mobili-
        zation During Suggestion of Exercise and Stress Using Hypno-
        sis and Sodium Amytal. Psychosomatic Medicine 35:5:367-374
        (1973).

190.   Horstman, D., Mendez, J., Buskirk, E.R., Boileau, R.,
        Nicholas, W.C., Lipid metabolism during heavy and moderate
        exercise. Medicine and Science in Sports 3:1:18-23 (1971).

191.   Felig, P., Wahren, J., Fuel homeostasis in exercise, N.
        England J. Med. 21:1978, 1975.

192.   Bizzi, A., and Garttini, S. Drugs lowering plasma free fatty
        acids: Similarities and dissimilarities with nicoltinic acid
        effect. Metabolic effects of Nicotinic Acid and its Deriva-
        tives. Edited by Gey, K.F. and Carlson, L.A. (1975).

193.   Carlson, L.A. Nicotinic acid: its metabolism and its effects
        on plasma free fatty acids. Metabolic Effects of Nicotinic
        Acid and its Derivatives. Edited by K. F. Gey and L.A.
        Carlson.(1971).

194.   Schliere, G. and Dorow, E., Dirurnal patterns of triglycer-
        ides, free fatty acids, blood sugar, and insulin during
        carbohydrate induction in man and their modification by noc-
        turnal suppression of lipolysis. J. Clin. Invest. 52:732
        (1973).

195.   Carlson, L.A. Nicotinic acid and inhibition of fat mobilizing
        lypolysis. Present status of effects on lipid metabolism.
        Advan. Exp. Molec. Biol. 109:225 (1978).

196.   Fuccella, L.U., Goldaniga, G., Lovisolo, P., Maggi, E.,
        Musatti, L., Mandelli, V., and Stirtori C.R. Inhibition of
        lipolysis by nicotinic acid and by acipimox. Clin. Pharmacol.
        Ther. 28:790 (1980).

197.   Kaijser, L., Elund, B., Olsson, A.G., and Carlson, L.A.
        Dissociation of the effects of nicotinic acid on vasodilation
        and lipolysis by a prostaglandin synthesis inhibitor,
        indomethacin, in man. From the Dept. of Clinical Physiology
        and Gustaf V. Research Institute, Karolinska Hospital, Stock-
        holm, Sweden.

198.   Nye, E.R. and Buchanan, H Short-term effect of nicotinic
        acid on plasma level and turnover of free fatty acids in
        sheep and man. Journal of Lipid Research 10:193 (1969).

Page 45

199. Carlson, L.A., Oro, L., Ostman, J. Effect of a single dose of nicotinic acid on plasma lipids in patients with hyperlipoproteinemia. Acta Med. Scand. 183:457 (1968).

200. Conner, W.E., Witlak, D.T., Stone, D.B. and Armstrong, J.S., Cholesterol balance and fecal neutral steroid and bile acid excretion in normal men fed dietary fats of different fatty acid composition. J. Clinic. Invest. 48:1363 (1969).

201. Shepherd, J., Stewart, J.M., Clark, J.G. and Carr, K., Sequential changes in plasma lipoproteins and body fat composition during polyunsaturated fat feeding in man. Br. J. Nutr. 44:265 (1980

202. Century, B., A role of the dietary lipid in the ability of phenobarbital to stimulate drug detoxification. J. Pharm. Exp. Therap. 185:185-194 (1973).

203. Effect of Certain Dietary Oils on Bile-Acid Secretion and Serum-Cholesterol. Lewis, B., The Lancet, 24 May, 1958.

204. Schnare, D.W., Robinson, P.C., Reduction of Hexachlorobenzene and Polychlorinated Biphenyl Human Body Burdens. International Agency for Research on Cancer, World Health Organization, Scientific Publications Series, Vol. 77, Oxford University Press.

205. Dewhurst, M., Gross, J.F., Sim, D., et al, The effect of rate of heating or cooling prior to heating on tumor and normal tissue microcirculatory blood flow, Biorheology 21 (4): 539-558, 1984.

206. Muller-Klieser, W., Vaupel, P., Effect of hyperthermia on tumor blood flow, Biorheology 21(4): 529-538.

207. Gey, K.F., Carlson, L.A. (eds.), Metabolic Effects of Nicotinic Acid and its Derivatives, Published by: Hans Huber Publishers, Bern, Switzerland.

208. Kaijser, L., Elund, B., Olsson, A.G., and Carlson, L.A. Dissociation of the effects of nicotinic acid on vasodilation and lipolysis by a prostaglandin synthesis inhibitor, indomethacin, in man. From the Dept. of Clinical Physiology and Gustaf v. Research Institute, KarolInska Hospital Stockholm, Sweden.

209. Eklund, B., et al., Prostaglandins, June, 1979. Vol. 17, No. 6.

Page 46

210. Vander, A.J., Nutrition, Stress and Toxic Chemicals. Ann Arbor: University of Michigan Press. 1981.

211. Smith, R.L., Implications of Biliary Excretion (Chapter 8), In: The Excretory Function of Bile, Published by Chapman and Hall, Ltd., London, 1973.

212. Smith, R.L., Chlorinated Hydrocarbon Pesticides (Chapter 16), In: The Excretory Function of Bile, Published by Chapman and Hall, Ltd., London, 1973.

213. Moore, R.B., Anderson, J.T. Taylor, H.L., Keys, A. and Frantz, Jr., I.D., Effect of Dietary Fat on the Fecal Excretion of Cholesterol and Its Degradation Products in Man. The Journal of Clinical Investigation: 47:1517-1534 (1968).

214. Hellman, L. Rosenfeld, R.S., Insull, Jr., W. and Ahrens, E.H., Intestinal Excretion of Cholesterol: A Mechanism for Regulation of Plasma Levels. J. of Clinic. Invest. 36:898 (1957).

215. Sodhi, H.S., Wood, P.D.S., Schlierf, G. and Kinsell, L.W., Plasma, Bile and Fecal Sterols in Relation to Diet, Metabolism 16:4:334-344 (1967)

216. Moore, R.B., Anderson, J.T. Taylor, H.L., Keys, A. and Frantz, Jr., I.D., Effects of Dietary Fat on the Fecal Excretion of Cholesterol and its degradation Products in Man. The Journal of Clinical Investigation: 47:1517-1534 (1968).

217. Conner, W.E., Witlak, D.T., Stone, D.B. and Armstrong, J.S., Cholesterol balance and fecal neutral steroid and bile acid excretion in normal men fed dietary fats of different fatty acid composition. J. Clinic. Invest. 48:1363 (1969).

218. Cooney, A.H., Pantuck, E.J., Hsiao, K-C, et al., Regulation of drug metabolism in man by environmental chemicals and diet. Fed. Proc. 36:1647-1652, 1977.

219. Century, B., A role of the dietary lipid in the ability of phenobarbital to stimulate drug detoxification, J. Phar. Exp. Therap. 185:185-194, 1973.

220. Meester, W, A progress report on the effect of polybrominated biphenyls (PBB) in Michigan residents. Vet. Human Toxicol. 22:2, 1980.

221. Richter, E., Lay, J., Klein, W. and Korte, F., Paraffin stimulated excretion of carbon-14 labeled 2,4,6,2',4'-pentachlorobiphenyl by rats. Toxicol. Appl. Pharmacal. 50:17-24, 1979.

222. Kimbrough, R., Burse, V. and Liddle, J., Toxicity of polybrominated biphenyl. Lancet, Sept. 17:602-3,-1977.

223. Stoewsand, G., Inhibition of hepatic toxicitys from polybrominated biphenyls and aflatoxin B in rats fed cauliflower. J. Environ. Pathol. Toxicol. 2:399-406, 1978.

224. Cohn, W., Boylan, J., Blanke, R., Fariss, J., Howell, J. and Guzelian, P, Treatment of chlordecone (Kepone) toxicity with cholestyramine: Results of a controlled clinical trial. N. Eng. J. Med. 298:243-248, 1978.

225. Wood, P., Shioda, R., and Kinsell, L., Dietary regulation of cholesterol metabolism. Lancet 2:604, 1966.

226. Kimbrough, R., Korver, M., Burse, V. and Groce, D., The effect of different diets or mineral oil on liver pathology and polybrominated biphenyl concentration in tissues, Toxicol. Applied Pharmacal. 52:442-453, 1980.

227. Innami, S., Nakamura, A., Miyazaki, M., Nagayama, S., and Nishide, E., Further studies on the reduction of vitamin A content in the livers of rats given polychlorinated biphenyls, J. Nutr. Sci, Vitaminol. 22:409-418, 1977.

228. Kato, N., Kato, M., Kimura, T., and Yoshida, A., Effect of dietary addition of PCB, DDT or HGT and dietary protein on vitamin A and cholesterol metabolism. Nutr. Rep. Int. 18: 437-445, 1978.

229. Chakraborty, D., Bhattacharyya, A., Chatterjee, J., Chatterjee, K., Sen, A., Chatterjee, s., Majumdar, K., and Chatterjee, G., Biochemical studies on polychlorinated biphenyl toxicity in rats: manipulation by vitamin C. Int. J. Vitam. Nutr. Res. 48:22-31, 1978.

230. Downing, D.T., Stewart, M.E., Strauss, J.S., Estimation of sebum production rates in man by measurement of the squalene content of skin biopsies. J. Invest. Derm. 77:358 (1981).

Page 48

231.   Cotterill, J.A., Cunliffe, W.J., Williamson, B., Variation in skin surface lipid composition and sebum excretion rate with time. Acta. Derm (Stockholm) 53:271 (1973).

232.   Kosugi, H.,Ucta, N. The Structure of Triglyceride in human sebum. Japan J. Exp. Med. 47:335 (1977).

233.   Wolff, M.S., Taffe, B., Boesch, R.R. and Selikoff, I.J., Detection of polycyclic aromatic hydrocarbons in skin oil obtained from roofing workers'. Chemosphere 11:595 (1982).

234.   Charnetski, W.A., Organochlorine insecticide residues in preen glands of ducks: Possibility of residue excretion. Bull. Envir. Cont. Toxicol. 12:672 (1974).

235.   Cunliffe, W.J., Buxton, J.L., and Shuster, S., The effect of local temperature variations on the sebum excretion rate. Br. J. Derm. 83:650 (1970).

236.   Williams, M., Cunliffe, W.J., Williamson, B., Forster, R.A., Cotterill, J.A. and Edwards, J.C., The effect of local temperature changes on sebum excretion rate and forehead surface lipid composition. Br. J. Derm. 60:53 (1973).

237.   Killum, R.E., Tochitani, Sh., and Strangfeld, K.J., Human sebaceous gland lipids in vitro incubations with 14-C-labelled compounds. Inves. Derm. 60:53 (1973).

238.   Downing, D.T., Strauss, J.S., Ramasastry, P., Abel, M., Lees, C.W., Pochi, P.E., Measurement of the Time Between Synthesis and Surface Excretion of Sebaceous Lipids in Sheep and Man. J. Invest. Dermatology 64:215-219 (1975).

239.   Downing, D.T., Strauss, J.S., Norton, L.A., Pochi, P.E., Stewart, M.E., The Time Course of Lipid Formation in Human Sebaceous Glands, J. Invest. Derm. 69:4:407-412 (1977).

240.   Henderson, G.L. and Wilson, B.K. Excretion of methadone and metabolites in human sweat. Res. Comm. Chem. Pathol. Pharmac. 5:1 (1973).

241.   Sunderman, F.W., Jr. Hohnadel, D.C., Evenson, M.A., Wannamaker, B.B., and Dahl, D.S. Excretion of copper in sweat of patients with Wilson's disease during sauna bathing. Ann. Clinic. Lab. Sci. 4:407 (1974).

Page 49

242. Hohmadel, D.C., Sunderman, Jr., F.W., Nechay, M.W., McNeely, M.D., Atomic absorption spectrometry of nickel, copper, zinc, and lead in sweat collected from healthy subjects during sauna bathing. Clin. Chem. 19:1288 (1973).

243. Emmett, E.A., Cohn, J.R., The excretion of trace-metals in human sweat. Ann. Clin. Lab. Sci. 8:270 (1978).

244. Howard, L.J., Marbach, R.I., Drug excretion in human eccrine sweat. J. Inves. Derm. 56:182 (1971).

245. Williams, M.L. and Elias, P.M. N-Alkanes in normal pathological human scale. Biochem. Biophys. Res. Comm. 107:322 (1982).

246. Schluneggar, U.P., Distribution patterns of n-Alkanes in human liver, urine and sweat. Biochim. Biophys. Acta. 260:339 (1972).

247. Uree, T.B., Muskens, A. Th., J.M. and VanRossum, J.M., Excretion of Amphetamines in human sweat. Arch. Int. Pharmac. 199:311 (1972).

248. Shields, D.O., The elimiation of lead in sweat. Australian Ann. Med. 3:225 (1954) Correc. 3:318.

249. Thaysen, J.H., Schwartz, I.L., The permeability of human sweat glands to a series of sulfonamide compounds. J. Exp. Med. 98:261 (1953).

250. Schnare, D.W., Ben, M., Robinson, P., Shields, M. Body Burden Reductions of PCBs, PBBs and Chlorinated Pesticides in Human subjects. Ambio, Vol. 13, No. 5 - 6 (1984).

251. Schnare, D.W., Robinson, P.C., Reduction of Hexachlorobenzene and Polychlorinated Biphenyl Human Body Burdens. International Agency for Research on Cancer, World Health Organization, Scientific Publications Series, Vol. 77, Oxford University Press.

252. Schnare, D.W., Denk, G., Shields, M., Brunton, s., Evaluation of a detoxification regimen for fat stored xenobiotics. Med. Hyp. 9:265 (1984).

253. Root, D.E. et al, Diagnosis and Treatment of Patients Presenting Subclinical Signs and Symptoms of Exposure to Chemicals Which Bioaccumulate in Human Tissue. Proceedings of the National Conference on Hazardous Wastes and Environmental Emergencies, May 14-16, 1985, Hazardous Materials Control Research Institute.

Page 50

254.   Roehm, D., Effects of a program of sauna baths and megavitamins on adipose DDE and PCB's and on clearing of symptoms of Agent Orange (diO in) toxicity, Clin. Res. 31(2):243a, 1983.

255.   Personal communication of Megan Shields, M.D. and Ziga Tret-jak, M.D., October, 1986.

256.   Personal communication of Megan Shields, M.D..

257.   Foundation for Advancements in Science and Education, "THC Research Update," February, 1983.

258.   Personal communication of Megan Shields, M.D..

259.   Laposata, E.A. and Lange, L.G., Presence of Nonoxidative Ethanol Metabolism in Human Organs Commonly Damaged by Ethanol Abuse, Science 231:497-499, 1986.

260.   Personal communication of Martin Dumain, December, 1986.

*   *   *   *

OPPORTUNITY KNOCKING!

We are certain that you see the benefits in Detoxination, and the fact that hundreds of thousands of people around the world have completed the protocol (either by the Hubbard Method or ours), should confirm that there is great interest in detoxifying xenobiotics.

In the next few years we will be developing an exciting opportunity for Naturopathic Doctors, Functional or Integrative Doctors, Chiropractors, Physical Therapists, EMTs, Wellness and Fitness Experts, and others to become trained and certified in Detoxination!

Certified *Detoxinicians* will be in demand as we develop our network of Detoxination Wellness Centers, licensees, and franchises over the coming years.

If you own your own healthcare facility or wellness/fitness center, you can also become a certified licensee and provide Detoxination Services in your own business. Soon a franchise opportunity will also become an option.

Be sure to inquire or register to be notified once we roll this transformative program out. Use our Contact form to indicate that you would like to get involved once we have everything in place.

ABOUT THE AUTHORS

David E. Root, M.D., M.P.H. – Curriculum Vitae

PRESENT POSITION

Medical Director, Sacramento Medical Group, PC, Sacramento, CA.

CERTIFICATIONS

Certified by the American Board of Preventive Medicine in Aerospace Medicine in 1972.

Certified by the American Board of Preventive Medicine in Occupational Medicine in 1983.

Certified by the FAA in December 1984 as an Aeromedical Examiner, and in 1987 as a Senior Aeromedical Examiner.

Certified by the Industrial Medical Council of the State of California as an Independent Medical Examiner, 1991-1993.

Certified by the Industrial Medical Council of the State of California as a Qualified Medical Evaluator, 1991-2003.

Certified by the Medical Review Officer Certification Council as a Medical Review Officer in 1993; recertified in 1998 and 2003.

Certified by the U.S. Department of Health and Human Services and the Drug Enforcement Administration to prescribe Suboxone and Subutex (buprenorphine), March 2005.

Recertified by the Medical Review Officer Certification Council as an MRO 1/28/10, expired 1/28/16, Certificate # 10-08603.

MEDICAL LICENSURE

State of California, June 17, 1965.

EDUCATION

Undergraduate Studies:

High school graduate, San Juan H.S., Blanding, Utah, 2004.

University of Utah, B.S. Degree in Psychology, 1958.

Medical School:

Wake Forest University School of Medicine, Bowman Gray Campus, Winston-Salem, NC, M.D. degree 1962.

Internship:

USAF Hospital, Wright-Patterson AFB, Dayton, Ohio, 1962-63.

Residency:

Johns Hopkins University School of Hygiene and Public Health, Master in Public Health, Baltimore, MD, 1970. Phase II and III, USAF School of Aerospace Medicine, Brooks AFB, Texas, July 1970-February 1972.

EXPERIENCE

July 1991 to Present:

Private practice limited to Chemical Detoxification and Occupational Medicine. Additional services include annual FAA Class I, II, and III physicals for corporate executives, pre-employment physical examinations, biological monitoring, pulmonary function, and out-patient injury care, including minor surgery. I voluntarily terminated my general practice and hospital privileges as of July 1, 1991 so that I could direct all my energy to my specialties of Chemical Detoxification and Occupational Medicine.

September 1981 to July 1991:

Solo private practice of Chemical Detoxification, Occupational Medicine, and General Practice. Private practice limited to Chemical Detoxification and Occupational Medicine. In the area of Chemical Detoxification, as Medical Director of HealthMed from 1983 to 2007, I treated toxic exposure cases with an emphasis on not only industrial and workplace exposures, but also on helping street drug and prescription drug abusers get off and stay off drugs. This included sample collection of subcutaneous adipose, skin lipids, and other tissues for analysis of chlorinated hydrocarbons, PCBs, halogenated volatiles, trace metals, other lipophilic toxicants, and eventual detoxification treatment to reduce the xenobiotic body burden.

Additional services included annual FAA Class I, II, and III physicals for corporate executives, pre-employment physical examinations, biological monitoring, pulmonary function, and out-patient urgent care, including minor surgery, are particularly emphasized.

October 1980 to July 1981:

Staff Physician at Doctors Medical Center, Sharonville, Ohio.

MILITARY SERVICE

USAF, 20 years active service as Chief Flight Surgeon and Senior Pilot, retired as full Colonel, October 1, 1980.

June 1978 to October 1980:

Chief Aeromedical Advisor to the USAF Life Support System Program Office, Air Force Systems Command, Wright-Patterson AFB, Dayton, Ohio. Advised the Life Support SPO on the medical aspects of new life support equipment such as helmets, oxygen masks, etc. Was responsible for the occupational medicine aspects of missile and aircraft fuels, such as hydrazine, UDMH, JP

4, etc. Had chemical defense program responsibility as well. Remained fully qualified as an Air Force Senior Pilot, frequently flying the T-37 twin-jet trainer. During this period I was also appointed Associate Professor, Department of Community Medicine, Wright State University, Dayton, Ohio.

January 1976 to June 1978:

Senior Medical Officer/Pilot, RAF Institute of Aviation Medicine, Farnborough, England (USAF/RAF Exchange Program Assignment). Had total responsibility for planning and carrying out the RAF medical flight test program at IAM in the Hawker Hunter aircraft. This involved flight testing of helmets, masks, and chemical warfare defense equipment designed to prevent chemical exposure to aircrews. Also carried out in-flight physiological experiments on pulmonary ventilation under high G forces, and many other flight test protocols.

July 1973 to December 1975:

Chief Occupational/Aerospace Medicine and Deputy Hospital Commander, Beale AFB, Marysville, CA. Was responsible for the medical operations of the SR-71 Recon aircraft. This involved providing primary medical care for the aircrews and their families, dealing with many occupational medical problems such as exposure to the special fuels, lubricants, and solvents used in the SR-71, as well as hazardous noise pollution from the jet aircraft. Maintained currency in the T-38 jet trainer in support of the SR-71.

July 1972 to July 1973:

Hospital Commander, USAF Hospital, Takhli, Thailand. Managed the hospital in the later stages of the Vietnam War, and was in charge of the Occupational and Flight Medicine sections. This included responsibility for the Medical Civic Action Program, which involved regular trips into the surrounding Thai villages to provide medical care to the villagers.

July 1969 to February 1972:

Residency in Aerospace Medicine. Phase I at Johns Hopkins University, Baltimore, MD, 1969-70, M.P.H. 1970. Phases II and III at Brooks AFB, Texas, 1970-72.

June 1969:

USAF terminated its involvement in the Manned Orbiting Laboratory Program when the program was moved to NASA. I then applied for, and was accepted into the Residency program in Aerospace Medicine.

May 1967 to July 1969:

Combat-ready F-100 fighter pilot, B Flight Commander, and squadron Flight Surgeon, 55th TFS, 20th TFW, RAF Wethersfield, England. This assignment was required to provide pilot-in-command experience before entering the MOL Astronaut training program.

July 1965 to May 1967:

Undergraduate Pilot Training at Moody AFB, Valdosta, GA; Advanced Flying Training in the F-100 at Luke AFB, Phoenix, AZ as part of the MOL Program. Served as Class Commander at Moody (Class 65-A), and was assigned as Class Flight Surgeon at both bases.

January 1965:

Selected to become a Pilot-Physician Astronaut with the USAF Manned Orbiting Laboratory (MOL) Program.

September 1963 to June 1965:

Assigned as Chief of Aerospace and Occupational Medicine at Beale AFB, Marysville, CA. This assignment was before the arrival of the SR-71 and involved support of two KC-135 air refueling squadrons and one B-52 squadron. Primary medical care of the aircrews and their families and occupational medical support of flying ops were the main duties.

July 1963 to September 1963:

Attended the Primary Course in Aerospace Medicine, School of Aerospace Medicine, Brooks AFB, Texas. Recipient of the Distinguished Graduate Award.

September 1956 to August 1957:

USAF Undergraduate Pilot Training, Aviation Cadet Class 58-H. After three years at college, I entered pilot training at Lackland AFB, Texas as an Aviation Cadet; took Primary Flight Training in the T-34 and T-28 aircraft at Spence Air Base, Moultrie, GA. Before I could begin Advance Training in the T-33, USAF changed the service commitment, which I refused to accept. I was separated and returned to the University of Utah in September 1957.

HONORS

Testified in a major court case, Paris, France, June 2009.

Co-Chair, Third International Conference on Human Detoxification, New York City, NY, September 2005.

Co-Chair, Second International Conference on Human Detoxification, Stockholm, Sweden, September 1997.

Presentation to the British House of Lords Select Committee on the Gulf War Syndrome: Detoxification Treatment and Results, May 1997.

Chair, First International Conference on Human Detoxification, Los Angeles, CA, December 1995.

Fellow, American College of Occupational and Environmental Medicine, 1987.

Fellow, Aerospace Medial Association, 1980.
Fellow, Royal Aeronautical Society, 1978.
Fellow, American College of Preventive Medicine, 1972.
MILITARY DECORATIONS
USAF

- Legion of Merit Medal
- Bronze Star Medal
- Merit Service Medal W/Dev
- Commendation Medal
- National Defense Service Medal

- Small Arms Expert Marksmanship Ribbon
- Longevity Service Ribbon W/4Dev
- Outstanding Unit Award

Republic of Vietnam Gallantry Cross W/Dev

- Vietnam Service Medal
- Vietnam Campaign Medal

Royal Air Force

- Queens's Commendation for outstanding service in the air, 1978.

ORGANIZATIONS & AFFILIATIONS

Associate Clinical Professor, Department of Community Medicine, Wright State University School of Medicine, Dayton, Ohio, December 1978-1981.

Vice-Chairman and Chairman-Elect, Associate Fellows Group, Aerospace Medical Association, 1979-1980.

Member, Program and Membership Committees of the Aerospace Medical Association, 1978-1981.

Member, American College of Occupational and Environmental Medicine.

Chapter Councilor, Phi Rho Sigma Medical Society, Wright State University, Dayton, Ohio, 1979-1981.

Member, Order of Daedalians, Member, Phi Delta Fraternity, and Member, Sacramento Rotary Club.

Member, Sacramento/El Dorado County Medical Society, California Medical Association, and American Medical Association.

Member, Sacramento/El Dorado County Medical Society Environmental Health Committee, October 1983 to present.

Member, Western Occupational and Environmental Medical Association.

Senior Associate, Foundation for Advancements in Science and Education, 1983-present.

Senior Member, Scientific Advisory Board, Foundation for Advancements in Science and Education, 1994-present.

Senior Member, Joint Ad Hoc Medical Society Task Force on Employment and Disability under the State Department of Rehabilitation, 1987-1991.

Elected and Ordained Elder, Carmichael Presbyterian Church, February 1996.

PUBLICATIONS & PRESENTATIONS

"Closed Ecological Systems Suitable for Space Flight", Research & Reviews, 1962. The Bowman Gray School of Medicine, Wake Forest University, Winston-Salem, NC.

"Inspiratory Flow and Pulmonary Ventilation in Mock Air Combat", paper presented – Aerospace Medical Association Meeting, 1977.

"Pressure Breathing for G Pretesting", presented – Aerospace Medical Association Meeting, 1978. Chaired one scientific session.

"New Directions in the Design of USAF Aircraft Oxygen Systems and Components", presented – Aerospace Medical Association Meeting, 1979.

"Advanced Aircraft Oxygen Systems", presented – semi-annual SAFE Association meeting, April 1979.

"A Survival Avionics System for the 1980s", paper presented – Aerospace Medical Association Scientific Meeting, Anaheim, California, May 1980.

"Hazards of Environmental Exposure and Chemical Detoxification Treatment", presented – California State Occupational Safety & Health Adm. inspectors of Northern California, Sacramento, CA, 1984.

"Diagnosis and Treatment of Patients Presenting Subclinical Signs and Symptoms of Exposure to Chemicals with Bioaccumulate in Human Tissue", presented – National Conference on Hazardous Wastes and Environmental Emergencies and sponsored by Hazardous Materials Control Research

Institute and the U.S. Environmental Protection Agency, May 1985. Cincinnati, OH.

"Reducing Toxic Body Burdens Advancing an Innovative Technique", Root, D., Anderson, J., Occupational Health and Safety, Vol. 11, No. 4, 1986.

"Radon Gas: Review of Current Studies on Household Detection and Health Effects", presented – Environment Health Committee of the Sacramento/El Dorado County Medical Society, October 15, 1986.

"Excretion of a Lipophilic Toxicant Through the Sebaceous Glands: A Case Report", Root, D., Lionelli, G., Journal Toxicol – Cut. & Ocular Toxicol, 6(1), 13-17, 1987.

"Responses to Environmental Exposures", presented – Roseville Hospital nursing staff as part of a continuing education program, April 29, 1988.

"Occupational Toxins", presented – Auburn Faith Hospital medical staff members as part of a continuing education program, September 6, 1988.

"First Do Not Harm; Diagnosis and Treatment of the Chemically Exposed", Chapter 4, Chemical Contamination and its Victims, Quotom Books, 1989.

"Xenobiotic Reduction and Clinical Improvements in Capacitor Workers: A Feasible Method", Tretjak, Z., Root, D.E., Tretjak, A., Slinik, R., Edmunson, E., Graves, R., and Beckmann, S.L.J., Environmental Science and Health, A25:731-751, 1990.

Daniel L. Root, CEO

Daniel Root has been an entrepreneur in the field of Information Technology for over 30 years. He became the Practice Manager of his father's medical practice, Sacramento Medical Group, in 2015 after serving four years as Controller.

After installing the first computer billing and practice management system in 1985, Dan was "volunteered" to undergo the original Hubbard Method of detoxification consisting of 4-5 program hours per day for thirty-three days. Despite the grueling schedule, Dan was amazed at the results. Not only did he have more energy and enjoyed more restful nights, his I.Q. tests, which were performed before and after the program, showed an improvement of 10 points, and his focus and concentration were greatly improved as well.

Dan and his wife Suzy adopted three biological sisters after failing to conceive naturally. In 2003 their first two adoptions finalized, and then late in 2005 they learned of a newborn biological sister that was placed in the foster system. In 2006, the Roots welcomed their third adopted daughter into the family. Due to their unusual adoption story, the Roots spent the next three years as a "poster family" for Sierra Forever Families, representing the adoption service at fund-raising events and on radio talk shows. Their family photo from Disneyland was published in magazines, newspapers, and newsletters. Dan went on to serve on the Sierra Forever Families' Board of Directors for six years, and was active on the Fund Development Committee.

His passion for sauna detoxification developed after Suzy underwent Radio Active Iodine (RAI) therapy for her hyperthyroidism condition without any improvement. Upon discovering that toxins and nutritional deficiencies were primary factors in Suzy's condition – and that detoxification could have prevented the destruction of

Suzy's thyroid and subsequent enslavement to the pharmaceutical industry – Dan committed himself to improving the quality of life and health of others through Detoxination.

Dan lives in the Sacramento, California, area with Suzy and their daughters.

Along with his producer, Jon Robert Quinn, Dan co-hosts *The Get Detoxinated Show*, a weekly radio talk show aired on KSAC, 105.5 FM.

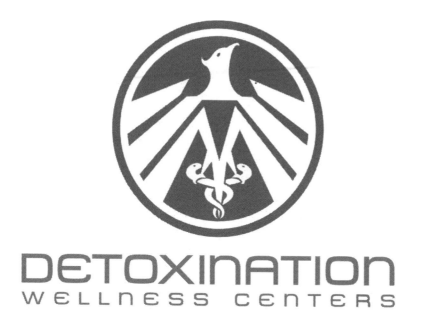

DETOXINATION
WELLNESS CENTERS

We're dedicated to improving your
quality of life and health by removing illness-
causing, fat-stored toxins, and promoting
non-toxic and organic lifestyle choices.

2706 Mercantile Drive
Rancho Cordova, CA 95742
(916) 366-0999
info@GetDetoxinated.com

www.GetDetoxinated.com

Index

Made in the USA
Middletown, DE
29 January 2019